A revised framework to address TB-HIV CO-INFECTION in the Western Pacific Region

WHO Library Cataloguing in Publication Data

A revised framework to address TB-HIV co-infection in the Western Pacific Region

1. Tuberculosis – complications. 2. Acquired immunodeficiency syndrome.
3. HIV infections – complications. 4. Western Pacific.

ISBN 978 92 9061 387 9   (NLM Classification: WF 200)

© World Health Organization 2008

All rights reserved.

The designations employed and the presentation of the material in this publication do not imply the expression of any opinion whatsoever on the part of the World Health Organization concerning the legal status of any country, territory, city or area or of its authorities, or concerning the delimitation of its frontiers or boundaries. Dotted lines on maps represent approximate border lines for which there may not yet be full agreement.

The mention of specific companies or of certain manufacturers' products does not imply that they are endorsed or recommended by the World Health Organization in preference to others of a similar nature that are not mentioned. Errors and omissions excepted, the names of proprietary products are distinguished by initial capital letters.

The World Health Organization does not warrant that the information contained in this publication is complete and correct and shall not be liable for any damages incurred as a result of its use.

Publications of the World Health Organization can be obtained from Marketing and Dissemination, World Health Organization, 20 Avenue Appia, 1211 Geneva 27, Switzerland (tel: +41 22 791 2476; fax: +41 22 791 4857; e-mail: bookorders@who.int). Requests for permission to reproduce WHO publications, in part or in whole, or to translate them – whether for sale or for noncommercial distribution – should be addressed to Publications, at the above address (fax: +41 22 791 4806; e-mail: permissions@who.int). For WHO Western Pacific Regional Publications, request for permission to reproduce should be addressed to Publications Office, World Health Organization, Regional Office for the Western Pacific, P.O. Box 2932, 1000, Manila, Philippines, fax: +632 521 1036, e-mail: publications@wpro.who.int

ACKNOWLEDGEMENTS

This document is a joint publication of STOP TB and the HIV/AIDS and STI Focus of the World Health Organization Regional Office for the Western Pacific.

Dr Kevin Cain, from the United States Centers for Disease Control and Prevention, is the leading author of the revised framework.

Dr Pieter van Maaren (STB), Dr Massimo Ghidinelli (HSI), Dr Philippe Glaziou (STB) and Dr Fabio Mesquita (HSI) are editors of the revised framework.

The following persons are acknowledged for their comments and contribution during the review process:

Alasdair Reid; Alumeci Tuivucilevu Taoi; Anna Marie Celina G. Garfin; Bernard Tomas; Chanta Chak; Chawalit Natpratan; Cheng Shiming; Christian Gunneberg; Connie Osborne; Cornelia Hennig; Dinh Ngoc Sy; Dominique Ricard; Dovdon Khandaasuren; Elsie Ryan; Esorom Daoni; Fuad Bin Hashim; Gaik Gui Ong; Gao Xing; Giampaolo Mezzabotta; Haileyesus Getahun; Hamizar Igbal Bin Abdul Halim; Han Trung Dien; Ikushi Onozaki; Jacques Sebert; Jadambaa Narantuya; Jamhoih Tonsing; Jay Varma; Josefa Koroivueta; Julian Elliott; Kamla Choumlivong; Kate Maree Learmonth; Katsunori Osuga; Khun Kim Eam; Liu Yuhong; Madeline Salva; Mao Tan Eang; Margaret Kal; Mary Ann Lansang; Masaki Ota; Massami Fujita; Mean Chhi Vun; Michael Voniatis; Murdorj Altankhuu; Nano Gideon; Nguyen Dac Vinh; Nguyen Thi Thanh Thuy; Nicole Seguy; Norio Yamada; Paison Dakulala; Paul Aia; Phouthone Southalack; Pilar Ramon-Pardo; Rajendra Yadav; Reuben Granich; Rosalind Vianzon; Samreth Sovannarith; Seng Sopheap; Shoko Sato; Tatsuo Sugiyama; Tran Van Son; Trinh Than Thuy; Wang Xuejing; Yoko Tsurugi; Zeenat Patel; Zhang Fujie.

LIST OF ABBREVIATIONS

AFB	acid-fast bacilli
AIDS	acquired immunodeficiency syndrome
ART	antiretroviral therapy
BCG	bacille Calmete-Guérin (vaccine against TB)
CPT	co-trimoxazole preventive therapy
DOTS	directly observed treatment, short-course
DST	drug-susceptibility testing
HIV	human immunodeficiency virus
IDU	injecting drug user
IPT	isoniazid preventive therapy
MDR TB	multidrug-resistant TB
MSM	men who have sex with men
OI	opportunistic infection
PCP	*Pneumocystis carinii* pneumonia
PITC	provider-initiated testing and counselling
PLWHA	people living with HIV/AIDS
PMTCT	prevention of mother-to-child transmission
STI	sexually transmitted infection
TB	tuberculosis
TST	tuberculin skin test
UNAIDS	Joint United Nations Programme on HIV/AIDS
UNODC	United Nations Office of Drugs and Crime
VCT	voluntary counselling and testing
WHO	World Health Organization
XDR TB	extensively drug-resistant TB

TABLE OF CONTENTS

ACKNOWLEDGEMENTS iii
LIST OF ABBREVIATIONS.. iv
TABLE OF CONTENTS v
EXECUTIVE SUMMARY vii
1. INTRODUCTION 1
2. BACKGROUND 3
3. CONCEPTUAL FRAMEWORK 11
4. TB-HIV SURVEILLANCE 17
5. HIV TESTING IN TB PATIENT CARE SETTINGS 21
6. INTENSIFIED TB CASE-FINDING IN HIV CARE SETTINGS 29
7. TREATMENT FOR PEOPLE WITH BOTH TB AND HIV 35
8. TB INFECTION CONTROL 39
9. TB-HIV CO-INFECTION IN CHILDREN 43
10. MONITORING AND EVALUATION 45
11. TB-HIV IN 'CLOSED SETTINGS' AND AMONG INJECTING DRUG USERS 47
12. COMMUNITY LEVEL TB-HIV COLLABORATION 51
13. PRIORITIES FOR PROGRAMMATICALLY RELEVANT RESEARCH 53

ANNEX

    ANNEX 1. COUNSELLING AND HIV TESTING USING ON-SITE STAFF 55
    ANNEX 2. HIV SURVEILLANCE AMONG TB PATIENTS WITH LOW BURDENS
                OF TB-HIV CO-INFECTION 61
    ANNEX 3. TB DATA FOR COUNTRIES IN THE WESTERN PACIFIC REGION........64
    ANNEX 4. DETAILS FOR CALCULATION OF INDICATORS 67

REFERENCES 71

EXECUTIVE SUMMARY

Tuberculosis (TB) is a leading cause of death and common presenting illness among people living with HIV. Likewise, HIV infection is more common among tuberculosis patients than among the general population. The consequences of failing to diagnose TB in a person living with HIV or of not diagnosing HIV in a TB patient are severe, as early mortality rates in people with both TB and HIV are very high.

In 2004, WHO developed a framework for TB-HIV control in the Western Pacific Region to address these intersecting epidemics. That framework called for increased HIV testing of TB patients, TB screening for people living with HIV, and appropriate medical treatment for persons with both tuberculosis and HIV, including antiretroviral therapy and co-trimoxazole preventive therapy. However, scaling-up of these activities has been slow. In 2006, just over 3% of TB patients in the Region were tested for HIV infection; the proportion of people living with HIV infection who were appropriately screened for TB is not known. Data from the Western Pacific Region and neighbouring countries reveal high mortality rates for people with both TB and HIV; rapid scaling-up of TB-HIV collaborative activities is urgently needed.

A revised framework is needed to properly address TB-HIV for several reasons: (1) scaling-up of activities has been too slow under the current framework; (2) recent data from the Region and neighbouring countries demonstrate that persons with both TB and HIV are very immunosuppressed at presentation and commonly die early; (3) efforts are needed to prevent TB transmission while scaling-up TB-HIV collaborative activities; (4) drug-resistant TB is an increasing problem among persons living with HIV, worldwide; and (5) expansion of TB laboratory services is needed to diagnose TB early in persons living with HIV, and to identify drug-resistant TB.

The previous framework relied largely on referral of patients between TB and HIV services to receive care. In order to avoid delays in TB and HIV diagnosis (and consequently unnecessary death), to avoid unnecessary exposure of people living with HIV infection to people with infectious TB, and to improve the uptake of HIV testing and TB screening, as well as appropriate medical treatment, this new framework attempts to avoid referral where possible by bringing the needed services to the patient. It proposes that people living with HIV should be screened for TB as part of their routine care at the facility they attend for HIV services. Similarly, it proposes that most TB patients and suspects should be offered HIV testing as part of routine TB diagnosis and care at the facility that diagnoses and/or treats their TB.

In addition to improving on the previous framework by addressing the barriers that have been identified since its introduction, this framework seeks to offer guidance to public health officials and their partners in dealing with the unique aspects of TB and HIV in the Western Pacific Region, including the varying HIV prevalence rates in countries throughout the Region and the greater importance of injecting drug use and commercial sex to the dynamics of HIV transmission in the Region.

1. INTRODUCTION

Worldwide, tuberculosis (TB) is a leading cause of death among people living with HIV and HIV is the most potent risk factor for the development of tuberculosis. People with both HIV and tuberculosis are likely to die far earlier than those HIV patients without tuberculosis. Likewise, TB patients with HIV infection are more likely to die earlier than TB patients who do not have an HIV infection. WHO's global response to TB-HIV co-infection includes the development of an interim policy on collaborative TB-HIV activities, with the aim of reducing tuberculosis transmission and decreasing the morbidity and mortality associated with co-infection.[1]

The Western Pacific Region carries up to one-third of the global TB burden and includes four of the 22 high-burden countries, but the HIV prevalence in most countries within the Region is far lower than that seen in sub-Saharan Africa.[2] Partly because of this distinction, the Western Pacific Region developed a regional framework for TB-HIV, which was published in 2004.[3] Since that time, access to antiretroviral therapy has expanded greatly within the Region, and some additional regional data about TB-HIV co-infection have become available. Unfortunately, the scaling-up of TB-HIV collaborative activities called for in the 2004 framework has been slow. As of 2006, just 3% of TB patients had been tested for HIV infection. No data are available regarding the scaling-up of TB screening for people living with HIV. Based on this, it is likely that many people with both TB and HIV are not being diagnosed in a timely manner.

Data about TB-HIV co-infection in the Western Pacific Region are limited. However, some have been published recently on co-infection in neighbouring countries, such as Thailand, which has similar TB and HIV epidemiology to that of countries in the Western Pacific Region. During the development of this revised framework, all available data were used, where possible, from the Region or neighbouring countries. Three aspects of the regional TB-HIV epidemiology described by these new data further demonstrate the need for revision of the current regional framework. First, using the previously recommended referral-based approach to TB-HIV collaborative activities, the proportions of TB patients tested for HIV infection and people living with HIV screened for TB in the Western Pacific Region are very low, and referrals between TB and HIV facilities may promote nosocomial transmission of TB as infection control is most often not implemented. Second, the case-fatality rate for persons with both HIV and TB is very high. Finally, most people in the Region with both HIV and TB tend to have advanced immune suppression at initial presentation.

Because of new policies and the new data about the epidemiology of TB-HIV in the Region, the Western Pacific Regional Office recognized that updates to the previous regional framework were needed. The goal of this updated framework is, therefore, to draw on global documents,[4,5] along with relevant recently published evidence, to improve TB-HIV control through the following primary means. First, national TB programmes and national AIDS programmes need to work collaboratively to decrease the case-fatality rate for persons with both TB and HIV through earlier detection of TB and HIV and appropriate management of people with both. Second, as one of the steps to achieve this, new approaches are needed to improve the rates of HIV testing among TB patients and of TB screening among people living with HIV. Third, TB laboratories must be expanded to meet the challenges of diagnosing TB and drug-resistant TB in people living with HIV. Finally, TB infection control measures must be scaled up to prevent transmission of disease within health facilities, a step made even more important in the era of multidrug-resistant (MDR) TB and extensively drug-resistant (XDR) TB.

While two separate epidemics can be successfully addressed through the efforts of two separate programmes focusing on each problem independently, containing epidemics that are as interrelated as TB and HIV requires close collaboration between the two programmes to achieve a common objective. This framework details the nature of the collaboration required to achieve this objective, including approaches to finding people with both TB and HIV through HIV testing of TB patients and TB screening of people living with HIV, appropriate interventions for TB-HIV patients and prevention of TB-HIV co-infection, and is designed to be useful for countries in the Region with different levels of HIV prevalence.

2. BACKGROUND

Tuberculosis

TB remains a major public health problem in the Western Pacific Region. In 2005, there were an estimated 3.6 million cases of TB (206 per 100 000 population), of which almost 1.9 million were new cases (110 per 100 000 population). Three countries (China, the Philippines and Viet Nam) accounted for about 90% of the total estimated new TB cases in the Region, with China alone accounting for 68%. In 2005, the regional case detection rate was 78% for new smear-positive cases and 63% for all forms of TB. In areas administering directly observed treatment, short-course (DOTS), the cure and treatment success rates were 87% and 91%, respectively, for the cohort of 566 237 new pulmonary smear-positive TB cases registered for treatment in 2004. Among the countries in the Region with a high burden of TB, only Papua New Guinea has a treatment success rate below the 85% regional target.[6] The 2005 data on TB notification, incidence and case detection in countries in the Western Pacific Region is shown in the table in Annex 3.

Along with HIV, another threat to TB control, both worldwide and in the Western Pacific Region, is drug-resistant TB. MDR TB, or TB that is resistant to both isoniazid and rifampicin, is also known to exist in the Region. In China, drug resistance surveys have been carried out in 13 of the 31 provinces; the proportion of new TB cases found to be MDR ranged from 2% (Hubei) to 10% (Liaoning). Meanwhile, Cambodia has reported that no new patients and 3% of re-treatment patients in a 2001 drug-resistance survey had MDR TB. In many other countries, current resistance patterns are unknown, although surveys are ongoing in some areas. The emergence of XDR TB worldwide has further increased the importance of good surveillance for drug resistance, as well as expansion of facilities to diagnose and treat MDR and XDR TB.

While smear microscopy has generally been widely implemented throughout the Western Pacific Region, TB culture and drug-susceptibility testing (DST) facilities remain limited. In addition, not all microscopy facilities are included in external quality assurance mechanisms.[7] Generally, it is estimated that to provide culture for diagnosis of paediatric, extrapulmonary and sputum-smear-negative HIV-infected TB, as well as DST for failure of category 1 and 2 treatments and contacts of MDR-TB cases, most countries will need one culture facility per 5 million population and one DST facility per 10 million population. However, for countries with large populations, one laboratory for culture and DST in each major administrative area may be sufficient.[8] Table 1 summarizes the coverage of laboratory services in selected Western Pacific Region countries, as of 2005.

TABLE 1. Coverage of laboratory services in selected countries in the Western Pacific Region, 2005.

Country	Population (thousands)	Access to diagnostic services						Laboratories included in EQA for microscopy	
		Sputum smear		Culture		DST			
		# of labs	Per 100 000 pop.	# of labs	Per 5 mil. pop.	# of labs	Per 10 mil. pop.	#	%
Cambodia	14 071	180	1.3	3	1.1	1	0.7	180	100
China	1 315 844	3060	0.2	125	0.5	47	0.4	2754	90
Lao People's Democratic Republic	5924	153	2.6	0	0	0	0	153	100
Mongolia	2646	35	1.3	1	1.9	1	3.8	35	100
Papua New Guinea	5887	60	1.0	1	0.8	0	0	5	8
Philippines	83 054	1858	2.2	3	0.2	3	0.4	491	26
Viet Nam	84 238	740	0.9	30	1.8	2	0.2	740	100

Pop = population
Mil = million
DST = drug-susceptibility testing
EQA = external quality assurance
Source: WHO Regional Office for the Western Pacific

HIV/AIDS

An overwhelming majority of the global HIV burden affects low- and middle-income countries, where 95% of people living with HIV reside. Of the global total of 33.2 million people living with HIV/AIDS at the end of 2007, 22.5 million (67.8%) were from sub-Saharan Africa, followed by 4.7 million (14%) from the WHO South-East Asia and Western Pacific Regions, 1.3 million of them in the Western Pacific Region.[9] In 2001, an estimated 0.75 million people were living with HIV/AIDS in the Western Pacific, thus the epidemic in the Region is still growing. However, overall HIV prevalence is still low, at about 0.1%. In 2007, an estimated 150 000 adults and children were newly infected and 63 000 AIDS deaths had occurred in the Western Pacific Region.[10] The HIV estimates for selected countries in Western Pacific Region are shown in Table 2.

TABLE 2. Latest HIV estimates in selected countries in the Western Pacific Region

Country	Year	Estimated number of people living with HIV/AIDS	Estimated HIV prevalence (age 15-49) (%)	Estimated AIDS deaths in 2005 (all ages)
Australia	2005	16 000	0.1	<500
Cambodia*	2006	65 000	0.9	10,000-12,000
China	2005	700 000	<0.1	31,000
Japan	2005	17 000	<0.1	1,400
Lao People's Democratic Republic	2005	3700	0.1	<100
Malaysia	2005	69 000	0.5	4,000
New Zealand	2005	1400	0.1	Na
Papua New Guinea*	2006	46 300	1.3	6,000**
Philippines	2005	12 000	<0.1	<1,000
Republic of Korea	2005	13 000	<0.1	<500
Singapore	2005	5500	0.3	<100
Viet Nam	2005	260 000	0.5	13,000

Source: AIDS epidemic update: 2006. Geneva, UNAIDS, 2006,
Except * Country consensus meetings
** Estimated data in 2007 using Spectrum software

Table 2 shows that the highest estimated HIV prevalence rates in the adult population (15-49 years) in the Region are found in Cambodia and Papua New Guinea. However, the absolute number of HIV-infected persons is highest in China, which accounts for about 700 000 people living with HIV infection, or half the regional total. High estimated numbers are also observed in Viet Nam, with 260 000 cases.

Although HIV prevalence in China is currently low, at approximately 0.05% in 2007, several provinces in central, southern and western parts of the country are facing serious, concentrated epidemics, spilling into the general population in some areas. Yunnan, Henan and Guangxi provinces are the worst affected, with over 30 000 cumulative HIV cases reported in 2005. Sexual transmission is now the main mode of HIV transmission. Of the estimated 700 000 people living with HIV at the end of 2007, 52% contracted HIV through sex, compared with 38% through injecting drug use. There are also indications of increasing HIV infection rates at antenatal sites. New HIV infections remain concentrated in populations with high-risk behaviours, including injecting drug users (IDU), sex workers and their clients, and men who have sex with men (MSM). Sexual transmission of HIV among migrant workers is also a concern given their potential to act as a bridging population to home villages and the general population.

Cambodia and Papua New Guinea have been categorized as having generalized epidemics (HIV prevalence >1% among the adult population aged 15-49). Cambodia is, however, showing a declining trend of HIV infection (revised prevalence rates from the peak of 2% in 1998 to 0.9% in 2006), while Papua New Guinea is showing an increasing trend (revised rates from 0.6 % in 2003 to 1.3% in 2006). In China, Malaysia and Viet Nam, the epidemics are concentrated in injecting drug users (HIV prevalence >5% among this group, but <1% among the adult general population nationally). The majority of countries in the Western Pacific Region, however, have low-level epidemics.

Unprotected heterosexual contact is the predominant method of HIV transmission in Cambodia, the Lao People's Democratic Republic, the Pacific island countries and areas, Papua New Guinea and the Philippines. HIV transmission related to injecting drug use is more common in those countries with a concentrated epidemic, as described above. Australia and New Zealand report that transmission there is more often among men who have sex with men. In general, HIV epidemics in countries in the Region have been driven largely by sex work and injecting drug use. HIV prevalence was estimated to be 17% among brothel-based sex workers in Cambodia in 2003,[11] and national surveillance data from Viet Nam provided an HIV prevalence rate of 31% among injecting drug users in Ha Noi in 2003.[12] It is becoming clear that men who have sex with men are also contributing substantially to Asian epidemics, although this population has been neglected for many years in the response to the epidemic.[13]

In the Western Pacific Region in 2007, the most recent data from low- and middle-income countries indicated that close to 90 000 AIDS patients were receiving ART (approximately 28% of the estimated number of people in need of treatment), representing a five-fold increase compared with about 16 000 patients in 2004.[14] The numbers of patients on ART in selected countries in the Western Pacific Regional in 2007 are shown in Table 3.

TABLE 3. Latest numbers of patients on ART in selected countries in the Western Pacific Region, 2007

Country	No. of ART sites	No. of people in need	No. of patients on ART	As of	% on ART
Cambodia	48	40 000	26 664	Dec 2007	67
China	1190	190 000	34 612	Dec 2007	19
Fiji	6	<200	28	Dec 2007	27
Lao People's Democratic Republic	2	<1000	700	Dec 2007	>95
Malaysia	171	20 000	6 590	Oct 2007	35
Mongolia	1	<100	3	Dec 2007	6
Papua New Guinea	38	5 900	2250	Dec 2007	38
Philippines	NA	1 100	336	Dec 2007	31
Viet Nam	202	67 000	14 969	Sept 2007	26
Western Pacific Region		320 340	89 231	Dec 2007	28

Source: Towards universal access: scaling up priority HIV/AIDS interventions in the health sector. Progress report 2008. Geneva, WHO-UNAIDS-UNICEF, 2008.
Notes: Need estimates generated using Spectrum software

TB-HIV co-infection

Background

HIV fuels the TB epidemic in several ways. HIV is the most powerful known risk factor for activation of latent TB infection to TB disease. The annual risk of developing TB in an HIV-infected person with TB infection ranges from 5% to 15%. Up to 50% of people living with HIV who are also infected with TB will develop TB disease during their lifetimes, compared with 5%–10% of HIV-uninfected persons.[15] The reported prevalence of latent TB infection in the Western Pacific Region is very high, up to 64% in Cambodia and 36% for the Region as a whole,[16] thus TB prevention and treatment is critical. Additionally, HIV increases the rate of recurrent TB, which may be due either to true relapse of treated disease or to re-infection.

TB also has an adverse effect on HIV progression and survival. Studies suggest that TB may increase HIV replication and may accelerate the natural progression of HIV infection.[17] In addition, people living with HIV who develop TB disease have a much higher case-fatality rate than those living with HIV without TB disease. TB is the leading cause of death among people living with HIV worldwide, with autopsy studies suggesting that up to 50% of HIV-related deaths are due to TB. [18,19,20]

Finally, at the level of immunodeficiency at which TB typically develops among patients in the Western Pacific Region, susceptibility to a range of other opportunistic infections (OI) is high. Many of these infections would be preventable through relevant prophylactic medications and the use of antiretroviral therapy to improve immune function.

Epidemiology of TB-HIV co-infection in the Western Pacific Region

Cambodia and Papua New Guinea report that up to 10% of new TB patients are HIV-infected countrywide. In other countries, including Viet Nam, some regions of the country report much higher rates of HIV infection than others. Table 4 shows the available data on HIV prevalence among TB patients in the Western Pacific Region. [21]

TABLE 4. Estimated HIV prevalence among newly notified TB cases in selected countries in the Western Pacific Region, 2005.

Country	HIV prevalence in newly notified TB cases (%)	Source and notes
Cambodia	10	*Comprehensive report on HIV/AIDS in Cambodia.* Phnom Penh, Ministry of Health, 2005. Note: estimated from a nationwide survey.
China	0.6	Estimated from the prevalence of HIV in the adult population, shown in Table 2, using methods described in: *Global tuberculosis control report 2007.* Geneva, World Health Organization, 2007: 12.
Lao People's Democratic Republic	0.6	
Malaysia	12.6	TB report to WHO. Ministry of Health, 2007. Note: 76% of new TB cases notified in 2005 were tested for HIV, of whom 12.6% tested positive.
Papua New Guinea	9.9	Estimated from the prevalence of HIV in the adult population, shown in Table 2, using methods described in: *Global tuberculosis control report 2007.* Geneva, World Health Organization, 2007: 12.
Philippines	<0.6	
Singapore	1.3	Ministry of Health (personal communication) 2007.
Viet Nam	4.2	TB Report to WHO. Ministry of Health, 2007. Note: obtained from the HIV sentinel surveillance system, not a representative estimate.

Source: *Tuberculosis control in the Western Pacific Region: 2007 report.* Manila, WHO Regional Office for the Western Pacific, 2007.

People with both TB and HIV in the Western Pacific Region tend to be more immunosuppressed and have higher case-fatality rates than those in sub-Saharan Africa. Published data suggest that the median CD4 count at diagnosis for people with both TB and HIV in sub-Saharan Africa is 186–393.[22,23,24] In contrast, the median CD4 count at diagnosis for people with both TB and HIV was reported to be 53-57 in Cambodia, Malaysia and Thailand.[25,26,27,28,29] These studies reflect a range of experiences, from a referral centre in Thailand to a rural clinic in Cambodia.[30,31] While a recent publication suggests that 24%-72% of people with both TB and HIV in sub-Saharan Africa have a CD4 count of <350 and thus qualify for ART if this threshold is used,[32] the above studies report that 88%-100% of people with both TB and HIV in the Western Pacific Region and Thailand had a CD4 count of <200. These findings are important for TB-HIV collaborative activities for two main reasons: (1) published estimates of the number of TB patients who will be eligible for ART may not be applicable to the Western Pacific Region if based on data from Africa; and (2) early diagnosis of both TB and HIV, along with early access to appropriate treatment for persons with both TB and HIV, is critical to saving lives.

Perhaps not surprisingly, given their very immunosuppressed presentations, people with both TB and HIV in Cambodia, Thailand and Viet Nam have much higher case-fatality rates than those in sub-Saharan Africa. Case-fatality is reported to be 26%-56% during TB treatment without ART, with up to half of all deaths occurring within two months.[33,34,35,36,37] This contrasts with case-fatality rates of 6%-39% reported in sub-Saharan Africa,[38] most below the range reported in Cambodia, Thailand and Viet Nam.

While data are not available for most countries in the Western Pacific Region, the available data have important implications for TB-HIV control in the Region. First, the high degree of immunosuppression and high early case-fatality rates among people with both TB and HIV mandates that co-infected people be diagnosed as quickly as possible. This will require improvements in current levels of HIV testing among TB patients and TB screening among people living with HIV, along with improvements in the quality of TB diagnosis. Second, the fact that almost all people with both TB and HIV in the Western Pacific Region have CD4 <200 suggests that finding these patients would be a high-yield approach to identifying people living with HIV who are eligible for ART. Finally, these data suggest that ensuring that all TB-HIV patients have early access to appropriate OI prophylaxis and ART is critical to decreasing case-fatality rates.

Current status of TB-HIV interventions in the Western Pacific Region

Available data on the current level of implementation of TB-HIV activities in the Western Pacific Region are not encouraging. Table 5 shows currently available data about implementation of TB-HIV activities in selected countries. The numbers may represent both an absence of activities and, perhaps even more, an absence of data. There is an urgent need to scale up activities where they are lacking and to increase monitoring and evaluation in all areas so that progress can be more accurately assessed.

TABLE 5. Proportion of TB patients tested for HIV and proportion of people with both TB and HIV receiving CPT and ART in selected countries in the Western Pacific Region, 2004-2005.

Country	Proportion TB patients tested for HIV (%)		Proportion of people with both TB and HIV receiving:			
			CPT (%)		ART (%)	
	2005	2006	2005	2006	2005	2006
Cambodia	2.9	10	?	?	?	?
China	?	0.14	?	?	?	?
Malaysia	?	81	?	?	?	?
Papua New Guinea	?	?	?	?	?	?
Viet Nam	?	15	?	?	?	?
Western Pacific Region	0.6	3.2	0.5	42	1.6	22

Source: Data presented here are the official data reported to WHO by member countries. *Global tuberculosis control: surveillance, planning, financing. WHO report 2007.* Geneva, World Health Organization, 2007.
? = Data not known or not reported.

3. CONCEPTUAL FRAMEWORK

Aims of the framework

The aims of the revised TB-HIV framework for the Western Pacific Region are shown in Box 1.

Countries should conduct TB-HIV surveillance that is appropriate to their local epidemiology. Since HIV prevalence among TB patients in the Region varies widely, this framework provides approaches to surveillance that are relevant to all situations.

Finding people with both TB and HIV is accomplished through HIV testing of TB patients and TB screening among people living with HIV. In this framework, one section is devoted to each of these topics. For HIV testing of TB patients, the recommended approach is provider-initiated HIV testing and counselling (PITC).[39] Initiating HIV testing at TB treatment facilities would increase the proportion of TB patients who are tested for HIV infection, decrease the time to HIV testing and treatment and thereby improve survival, and improve infection control by not exposing persons at HIV testing centres, many of whom are HIV-infected, to infectious TB patients.

> **Box 1.** Aims of revised TB-HIV framework
>
> - Conduct TB-HIV surveillance that is appropriate for the epidemiological situation of the country.
> - Diagnose people with both TB and HIV as early as possible through early HIV testing of TB patients and TB screening of people living with HIV.
> - Ensure that people with both TB and HIV have early access to life-saving treatment, including antiretroviral therapy and opportunistic infection prophylaxis.
> - Improve infection control at TB and HIV care facilities to decrease the potential for the spread of TB among highly susceptible persons.
> - Prevent new cases of HIV and TB.

Improving TB screening and diagnosis of HIV patients require improvements in both the quantity of patients screened and the quality of screening / diagnosis. All people living with HIV should be screened for TB (1) at the time of HIV diagnosis, (2) before starting antiretroviral therapy, and (3) at each follow-up visit.[40] The capacity to screen patients for TB should be fully established within all public health facilities designated to provide ART in order to avoid delays in diagnosis. To improve the quality of screening, evidence-based diagnostic algorithms should be used. In addition, facilities for chest radiography and TB laboratory services, including solid and liquid culture,[41,42] should be scaled up in order to improve the sensitivity of TB diagnosis for cases in which additional diagnostic testing is needed, and also to facilitate the diagnosis of drug-resistant TB.

Since most people with both TB and HIV are very immunosuppressed at the time of diagnosis in the South-East Asian countries of the Western Pacific Region, almost all will be eligible for ART immediately according to the criteria used in countries throughout the Region. In addition, their advanced levels of immunosuppression make these patients susceptible to a wide range of other OI. Appropriate measures should be in place to ensure that people with both TB and HIV, once identified, have early access to clinics that provide both ART and OI prophylaxis.

In order to decrease TB transmission at HIV diagnosis and care facilities, efforts to improve infection control are needed. A stronger focus on PITC for the diagnosis of HIV infection in TB patients will decrease the need to send infectious TB patients to HIV testing facilities for diagnosis. Since ART is typically not provided in TB treatment facilities, HIV treatment facilities will routinely have a mix of people living with HIV, with and without TB disease. Thus, such facilities should implement infection control measures. Finally, specialized TB treatment facilities that provide care for multidrug-resistant TB should also develop the capacity to manage antiretroviral therapy, to avoid sending MDR TB patients to HIV treatment facilities and exposing susceptible patients to drug-resistant TB.

Finally, scaling-up of HIV and TB prevention efforts is needed. People living with HIV who are screened for and found not to have TB should be evaluated for IPT. At the same time, HIV prevention messages should be provided to TB patients. This can include general messages about HIV prevention, since many TB patients practise HIV risk behaviours, such as intravenous drug use or unprotected sex. Additionally, TB patients who test negative for HIV infection can be advised about how to prevent such infection, while TB patients who test positive for HIV infection should receive further counselling about prevention of transmission. This counselling can take place at the clinic to which they are referred for HIV treatment.

The general approach to HIV testing of TB patients, TB screening of people living with HIV, and treatment of people with both TB and HIV is shown in Figure 1.

Approach to implementation

The foundation of TB-HIV activities is successful joint planning, collaboration and oversight between the HIV programme and the TB programme at all levels, from the national level down to the health facility and community. As part of this process, both programmes should jointly identify the roles and responsibilities of each with respect to financing and accountability.

> **Box 2.** Key responsibilities of the national TB-HIV coordinating body
>
> - Establish a regular schedule for meetings.
> - Decide on a structure for subnational and facility-level oversight of TB-HIV activities.
> - Using this framework and taking account of local epidemiology, select appropriate policies and practices for each part of the country.
> - Design a plan for scaling-up of activities countrywide.
> - Procure and manage supplies (including, but not limited to supplies for HIV testing, chest radiography, sputum-smear microscopy, isoniazid, antiretroviral drugs).
>   - Determine who will procure each and how to procure each.
>   - Use epidemiology and historical consumption data to determine the amounts needed.
> - Advise on data management tools and process and design a system for joint monitoring and evaluation and supervision.

A TB-HIV coordinating body should be established at the national level for national TB-HIV planning and for overseeing implementation of joint activities. This group should have regularly scheduled meetings and should include the director (or a designee with decision-making authority) and additional members from each programme. Representatives of institutional partners, international agencies and support groups of people living with HIV/AIDS (PLWHA) may also be included. In addition, other sectors, such as the legal sector and other groups involved with injecting drug users and other 'closed settings', may be included. Suggested terms of reference for the national TB-HIV coordinating body are shown in Box 2. One approach that has been used successfully by some countries in the Western Pacific Region is to have a smaller group under the coordinating body that meets frequently to focus on technical issues.

Subnational and facility-level oversight

At the subnational level (regional, provincial or district), countries may elect to have a TB-HIV committee or just to appoint a TB-HIV focal person to join, where appropriate, existing coordination bodies in order to secure linkages with other ongoing programmatic activities. For example, some countries have provincial committees coordinating all HIV/AIDS interventions, including HIV testing, treatment and care, as well as home/community-based care. TB-HIV can become an element addressed by such a committee. In addition, each health facility should designate at least one TB-HIV focal person. All designated HIV treatment facilities should appoint a TB focal person, and likewise all TB treatment facilities should appoint an HIV focal person. TB-HIV focal persons should be responsible for facilitating local implementation. Oversight of local implementation can be provided by the district or provincial TB-HIV leadership.

Selecting appropriate policies and practices for local implementation

This framework highlights several areas in which joint planning and implementation are important. Sections of the framework on HIV testing of TB patients and TB screening of people living with HIV offer different options for implementing TB-HIV activities, and the general activities are shown in Figure 1. Different countries may choose to select different options, and multiple options may be needed within each country. These options should be selected by the coordinating body based on local epidemiology and local resources.

Plan for national scaling-up

Generally, it will not be possible to implement all the activities in this framework at one time. The national coordinating body should design a plan for scaling-up that: (1) implements activities as quickly as possible, in recognition of the current very high case-fatality rates in the Western Pacific Region; (2) ensures a high quality of services; and (3) uses local epidemiology to prioritize places most in need for scaling-up.

Procurement and supply management

In order to ensure that life-saving activities are duly supported by regular supplies, careful planning is needed. Epidemiology should be used to estimate:

(1) how many TB patients will be tested for HIV infection;

(2) how many people living with HIV will be screened for TB, and at what frequency:
 (a) the proportion that will need chest radiography;
 (b) the proportion that will need sputum-smear microscopy; and
 (c) the proportion that will need additional testing, including TB culture;

(3) the total number of people with both TB and HIV expected, and thus:
 (a) the amount of co-trimoxazole preventive therapy (CPT) needed for people with both TB and HIV; and

(b) the amount of alternative ART regimens needed for people with both TB and HIV; and

(4) the number of people living with HIV expected to need isoniazid preventive therapy (IPT).

Data management (monitoring and evaluation) and supervision of activities

The nature of monitoring and evaluation as regards TB-HIV activities is that data must be collected from both HIV and TB facilities (these include any facility that provides treatment for HIV or TB, which may include prisons health facilities or, potentially, clinics that treat sexually transmitted infections). Most of the key elements will be collected in the revised TB recording and reporting system. To accomplish this, TB and HIV programmes can engage in joint visits to sites, or a TB-HIV focal person can collect information from both the TB facilities and HIV facilities in a given area. This will facilitate accurate measurement of data. Details about the data that should be collected are available in section 9.

Similarly, many activities have both TB and HIV components. As such, the two programmes may want to consider joint supervisory visits in order to ensure that collaborative activities are being properly implemented according to the national plan and guidelines.

FIGURE 1. Flow diagram for HIV and TB diagnosis and treatment

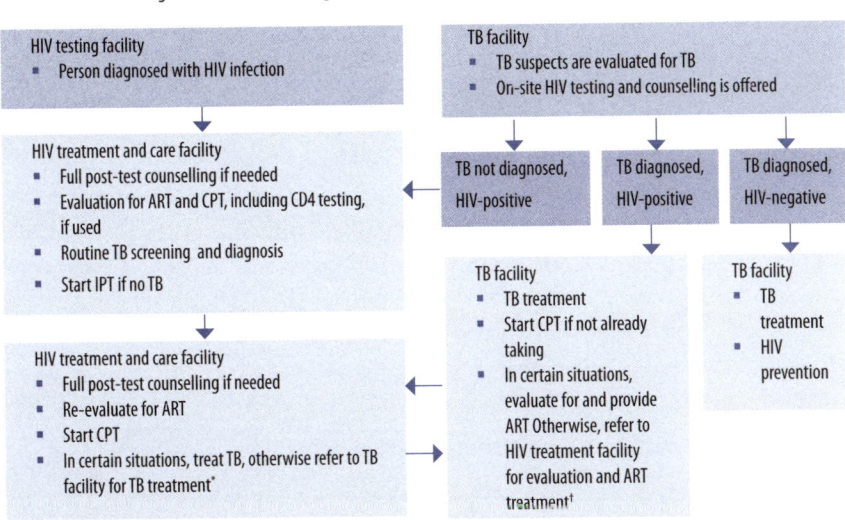

* TB treatment can be provided at the TB facility nearest to the patient's home or at the ART treatment facility, depending on the needs of the patient and the decision of the national programmes.

† ART treatment will generally be provided at the ART treatment facility. However, for patients with MDR or XDR TB, ART should be provided at the TB treatment facility. As capacity for MDR and XDR TB treatment is increased, provisions should be made to provide ART at these facilities as well, preferably by training staff at those facilities in ART use.

4. TB-HIV SURVEILLANCE

The importance of surveillance for HIV infection among tuberculosis patients has become increasingly recognized as the HIV epidemic has continued to fuel the TB problem and as new solutions have emerged to address this situation. A good overview of HIV surveillance among TB patients is provided in a WHO publication called *Guidelines for HIV surveillance among tuberculosis patients*.[43]

Surveillance activities for HIV usually refer to the intentional collection of data, through surveys, for example. However, it is increasingly recognized that surveillance systems can also make use of data that results from other activities where surveillance is a secondary objective. HIV surveillance data may thus be obtained from activities such as provider-initiated testing and counselling. However, the use of these routine data for the purposes of surveillance is only valid if HIV testing is sufficiently common that the routine data are representative of the population.

TB-HIV surveillance is, in general, not different from surveillance for other diseases and infections. However, surveillance methods must be adapted because of the wide variation in the prevalence rates of HIV infection and the importance of such issues as anonymity and confidentiality.

Rationale for surveillance

The overall objective of any communicable disease surveillance system is to collect, analyse and disseminate accurate epidemiological data that will inform public health programmes. This should contribute to a better understanding of the magnitude of the problem and provide reliable, timely and cost-efficient information for action.

It is important for national TB control programmes to determine and monitor the prevalence of HIV infection in TB patients over time, since this will provide a direct measure of the impact of the HIV epidemic on the tuberculosis problem. Surveillance is a useful tool for evaluating the current situation and for predicting future changes in TB incidence. Surveillance of TB-HIV is the starting point for intensified case detection and for implementation of TB-HIV interventions. In some countries, surveillance data may be used to develop a phased approach to implementation of activities, such that regions with the greatest need are prioritized for early implementation. Likewise, surveillance in countries with low

HIV prevalence can be used to determine whether a certain threshold level of HIV prevalence has been reached.

Surveillance methods

The appropriate method(s) for the surveillance of HIV among tuberculosis patients depends on the HIV epidemic state of each individual country and on the proportion of TB patients who are tested for HIV infection as a part of routine care. There are three main surveillance methods: periodic surveys, sentinel surveillance and data from routine care.

Periodic surveys

Periodic seroprevalence surveys are the main surveillance method for measuring HIV prevalence among tuberculosis patients in many countries around the world. In countries without information on the magnitude of HIV prevalence among TB patients, a survey is the preferred method. Well-conducted, cross-sectional seroprevalence surveys, using a representative sample of tuberculosis patients, can provide reliable estimates of HIV prevalence among tuberculosis patients.

Careful consideration of ethical issues is needed when planning a seroprevalence survey. In general, a survey that includes HIV testing should provide test results and post-test counselling to those tested, and should offer referrals to care for those with a positive test result. This approach is ethically preferable to unlinked, anonymous HIV testing, where specimens collected for a different purpose are tested for HIV with no link to the patient's name or identifying information and thus no opportunity to provide results.

Sentinel surveillance

Sentinel surveillance can be described as the system by which "specific sites and population groups are selected, a predetermined number of persons are routinely tested, and testing is performed in a regular and consistent way".[44] When interpreting results from surveys using sentinel methods, it is important to estimate, first, the extent to which the people tested are representative of the sentinel population from which they are drawn and, second, the extent to which the sentinel population is representative of the general tuberculosis population. In general, sentinel methods do not provide data representative of a whole country and even trends within sentinel sites should be interpreted with caution as the catchment population of a site may vary over time. Therefore, sentinel surveillance should be calibrated every three to five years using cross-sectional surveys.

In addition, sentinel surveillance methods can be used for surveillance in populations that may be missed by other methods, including intravenous drug users and prisoners. Since these groups have been an important part of the HIV epidemic in the Western Pacific Region, and since localized epidemics in these populations can grow rapidly if not addressed early, surveillance should specifically target these populations.

Data from routine care

Data from routine patient care may be collected through a variety of methods. In general, the methods used to capture data from routine care will largely depend upon the existing tuberculosis and HIV/AIDS programmes in a country, as well as the resources available for surveillance activities. However, data from routine patient care should be based on the routine reporting of all individuals with tuberculosis who are tested for HIV infection, whether in the setting of a voluntary counselling and testing (VCT) site or as part of PITC.

Implementation of surveillance

As mentioned above, in situations where the prevalence of HIV in TB patients is unknown, a baseline survey may need to be conducted. In other situations, the preferred surveillance method should be the use of data from routine care. However, it must be emphasized that data from routine care will only reflect the prevalence of HIV infection among TB patients accurately when the uptake of HIV testing is high.

At times, an extremely accurate estimate of HIV prevalence among TB patients is not necessary, but rather, a determination is needed regarding whether a certain threshold has been met (i.e. 1% HIV prevalence in TB patients). Routine data can be used to determine a low-end estimate of HIV prevalence among TB patients, which may suffice for this situation. To do this, the total number of known people with both TB and HIV during a given time period should be divided by the total number of TB cases reported during the same time period. This will underestimate prevalence, as it essentially counts all untested persons as HIV-uninfected. However, if the goal is to determine whether prevalence exceeds a certain level, and if the low-end estimate exceeds that level, then no further data would be needed to address the question.

When routine data are not sufficient to make the appropriate public health decision, efforts should focus on increasing the proportion of TB patients tested for HIV infection and using these data once uptake is sufficiently high. In the interim, periodic surveys or sentinel surveillance should be used, and such surveys should be planned jointly by the national TB-HIV coordinating body. In some countries, this type of survey can be integrated into larger TB- or HIV-related surveys.

HIV prevalence among TB patients in some countries in the Western Pacific Region is very low. In these cases, for a survey to have sufficient power to provide a precise estimate of HIV prevalence among TB patients, the sample size would need to be very large. However, such precision is not necessary. Instead, surveys in such countries can be powered to reliably demonstrate that the prevalence is <1%. The sample size required for achieving this is much smaller, and this is suitable for making appropriate programmatic decisions.

Whichever surveillance method is used, it is important that sufficient attention is given to sampling, quality of laboratory procedures, data management and regular evaluation of the surveillance system. More detailed information on surveillance methods and methodological issues is provided in *Guidelines for HIV surveillance among tuberculosis patients*.[45]

Surveillance for tuberculosis among people living with HIV

While surveillance for HIV-infection among TB patients is widely practised around the world, including in some areas of the Western Pacific Region, surveillance for TB in people living with HIV is usually overlooked. However, the prevalence of TB disease among patients newly diagnosed with HIV infection is extremely high in the Region, up to 25%-43%.[46,47] It is important for national AIDS programmes to determine and monitor over time the prevalence of TB in newly diagnosed people living with HIV, as this is the most direct measure of the impact of the TB epidemic on the HIV programme. Such data can be used to plan the appropriate availability of specific TB diagnostic techniques in certain areas, including TB culture, procurement of appropriate antiretroviral therapy for TB-HIV patients, and infection control.

At this time, no country in the Western Pacific Region has sufficient data to rely on routine data to address this issue. In most cases, the prevalence of TB among newly diagnosed people living with HIV is not known, so a periodic survey would be the appropriate choice. Sentinel surveillance may also be appropriate in certain situations. Regardless of the method chosen, careful consideration should be given to laboratory procedures. Since many people living with HIV with TB disease have negative sputum smears, TB culture would be essential to give an accurate estimate of TB prevalence.

5. HIV TESTING IN TB PATIENT CARE SETTINGS

> **Box 3.** Key points for HIV testing in TB patient care settings
>
> - To the greatest extent possible, HIV testing should be made available to TB patients on site (at the facility where they are being treated for TB) to increase access and uptake.
> - HIV testing and counselling should be promoted in line with the WHO-recommended policy on provider-initiated testing and counselling.*
> - All TB patients should be tested for HIV infection.
> - HIV testing is needed for patients cared for by a variety of programmes (e.g., STI, PMTCT, TB). As such, testing in a facility should be available for patients from all programmes, and plans for scaling-up should be designed to meet the needs of all programmes.
>
> *Guidance on provider-initiated HIV testing and counselling in health facilities.* Geneva, World Health Organization, 2007.

HIV testing is recommended for all TB patients and suspects, because prevalence is higher in these populations than in most other groups and they can benefit early from life-saving interventions to prevent the high early case-fatality rate for people with both TB and HIV, which is particularly problematic in the Western Pacific Region.

Historically, the most widely practised method for accomplishing this has been to refer TB patients to an HIV testing facility for counselling and testing. Such facilities, often referred to as VCT sites, are designed to offer walk-in counselling and testing for persons who desire a test. This 'client-initiated' model of testing and counselling usually emphasizes individual risk assessment and management by counsellors, and involves lengthy pre-test counselling.[48]

After years of experience using this model, there is now substantial evidence to demonstrate that, on its own, it does not meet the needs of TB patients. The uptake of testing in the Western Pacific Region, which relies heavily on this approach, is very low. In 2004, only 0.7% of TB patients in the Region were tested for HIV infection; that number was 0.6% in 2005.[49] In Cambodia, the national AIDS programme has demonstrated that intensive efforts to refer patients can improve results; testing at sites where such efforts were focused, including support of patient transportation, showed that HIV testing of TB patients increased to 40%, a substantial increase over previous levels. However, testing rates levelled off at that point.

Most of Africa also initially relied on the referral approach, testing just 2% of TB patients for HIV infection in 2004.[50] However, as countries recognized that patients were often unable to access needed testing, they added additional testing options for TB patients. These options complemented the traditional approach by making it possible for TB patients to choose to be tested for HIV infection without referral to a specialized testing facility. Such options are often referred to as 'provider-initiated testing and counselling', or PITC.[51] In the WHO African Region overall, HIV testing among TB patients had increased to 11% by 2005. In countries that have implemented PITC, however, reported testing rates are substantially higher. Rwanda and Kenya, which have both implemented PITC, report that the proportions of TB patients tested for HIV infection were 81% and 64%, respectively, in the third quarter of 2006.[52] PITC has been demonstrated to be feasible in other countries with limited resources, as well as in countries in and near the Western Pacific Region, including Thailand and Viet Nam.[53]

Data from the Western Pacific Region support the conclusion that patients are less likely to be tested when on-site testing is not available. In Cambodia, under the referral approach, even when transportation to the nearest VCT site was supported, staff were trained and substantial resources were provided, only 47% of TB patients treated at facilities without VCT were tested, compared with 76% at facilities with on-site VCT.[54] This raises concerns about inequitable access to care, as poor patients who are unable to give up a day's wages or miss work for other reasons are less likely to be able to access testing. Data from Zambia suggest that rates of HIV testing are better under a PITC-based model, where the TB staff provide HIV testing, compared with even an on-site VCT-based approach. [55]

Even for those cases in which a designated testing facility is available within the hospital or health facility complex or very nearby, sending patients who are confirmed as having TB or who are TB suspects there unnecessarily exposes people living with HIV at the testing facility to TB, when the patients could be tested for HIV infection on site, thereby avoiding this exposure. This problem is further aggravated by the emergence of drug-resistant TB, for which case-fatality rates are even higher.

Available options for HIV testing of TB patients

PITC is the recommended approach for ensuring HIV testing and counselling for all newly diagnosed TB patients and suspects. To support its implementation, minimize discomfort for patients and clients, and address actual and potential barriers, WHO recommends systematic use of rapid tests, aiming for a 'same-day result' in the provision of HIV testing and counselling services.

There are several options for PITC implementation in TB settings, whereby PITC components (pre-test information, laboratory testing, post-counselling) could take place at different facilities. These options are summarized in Table 7. As discussed above, referring TB patients to a testing facility causes unnecessary exposure of people living with HIV to TB disease and, when the facility is not located near the DOTS site, uptake is also low. Efforts to provide testing without the need to refer the patient to another site are therefore preferred.

TABLE 7. Potential approaches to HIV testing of TB patients

	Approach 1	Approach 2	Approach 3
Pre-test information	At the DOTS site	At the DOTS site	At the DOTS site
HIV testing	At the DOTS site*	Patient sent to on-site HIV testing laboratory	Blood sent to on-site or off-site HIV testing laboratory
Test result and post-test counselling	At the DOTS site*. Patients with a positive result receives complete post-test counselling at the HIV treatment facility	At the DOTS site. Patients with a positive result receives complete post-test counselling at the HIV treatment facility	At the DOTS site. Patients with a positive result receives complete post-test counselling at the HIV treatment facility

* When approach 1 is used, a trained staff member based at the DOTS site can do the HIV testing and the post-test counselling or a mobile counsellor, who can visit several DOTS sites, can provide these services, especially if the workload at each site is very low.

Potential approaches to HIV testing among TB patients include three main options: (1) HIV testing and counselling provided at the DOTS site. (This can either be done with staff who are based at the site, or mobile counselling and testing could be employed, where a trained counsellor regularly goes to the DOTS clinic to offer HIV testing and counselling on site.); (2) following pre-test information in the DOTS facility, the patient could go to an on-site laboratory for blood collection and testing; and (3) following pre-test information and blood collection at the TB treatment site, blood specimens could be referred to the laboratory for HIV testing (in some cases, the laboratory may be at the HIV testing facility). In each of these approaches, any patient with a positive test result would be referred to the HIV treatment facility for complete post-test counselling and HIV care.

Mobile counselling and testing has been used successfully in some countries. The advantages of this approach include the need for a modest number of staff, which makes training, supervision and quality assurance more manageable, and provision of an on-site testing option for the patient, which should increase the uptake of testing and decrease the exposure of people living with HIV at the HIV testing facility to infectious TB patients. The disadvantages include the need for staff transportation, the need to visit each facility very frequently (e.g. once per week) to ensure that patients are diagnosed early, and the possibly very heavy client load, since all TB patients and suspects seen during the time since the previous visit would need to be seen on the same day. Finally, many individuals would have to return to the clinic for testing at a later date, which may result in drop-outs.

Collecting and testing blood at the DOTS facility has become a feasible approach to HIV testing due to the introduction of sensitive, specific, simple-to-use rapid antibody tests that do not require sophisticated laboratory services, running water or electricity. Testing can occur outside the laboratory setting, does not require specialized equipment, and can be carried out in primary health facilities by appropriately trained non-laboratory personnel, including counsellors and TB staff.[56]

The advantages of counselling and testing being carried out by staff at the DOTS facility, with or without the use of an on-site HIV testing laboratory (approaches 1 and 2 in Table 7), include:

- the immediate availability of services, thereby decreasing the number of drop-outs and diminishing delays;
- the provision of a testing option for the patient that does not require travel to another location (This should increase the uptake of testing and decrease the exposure of people living with HIV at the HIV testing facility to infectious TB patients.);
- the fact that there is no need for return visits for HIV testing;
- the distribution of testing across more sites, thus avoiding overloading of sites that serve multiple facilities; and
- the ability to integrate easily into the existing network of testing facilities by sending blood specimens to the same laboratory, thus simplifying supply and quality assurance.

The disadvantages include the need to train a larger number of individuals and to have a greater number of facilities, which will need supplies, quality assurance and appropriate supervision.

It should be emphasized that, regardless of the approach selected, WHO and UNAIDS do not support mandatory or coercive testing. All patients should have the option to refuse testing.[57]

Training

Regardless of the option chosen, selected providers will need to be trained in HIV counselling and testing. Training needs for TB providers differ from those for VCT counsellors. The information provided by TB staff before testing is much shorter and more focused. Training for PITC counselling also need not be as comprehensive. TB providers should be expected to provide pre-test information and post-test counselling for patients with a negative test result, and should be able to deliver a positive test result to a patient in a sensitive manner, with appropriate information, and to ensure that the patient is referred to an HIV treatment facility for full counselling and initiation of care. In some cases, providers will also need to be taught how to perform the test. Training materials designed to meet these needs in a four-day course are available online,[58] and these materials have been adapted and used as a three-day course to train TB staff in Thailand and Viet Nam on how to conduct counselling and perform the laboratory test. Less time may be needed for TB staff who do not need to learn how to perform the test.

Who should be tested?

Consistent with global guidance, and regardless of the type of epidemic present in the country (generalized, concentrated or low-level), HIV testing is recommended for all adults, adolescents and children presenting with signs, symptoms or medical conditions that could indicate HIV infection, including tuberculosis patients and suspects.[59] Failure to recommend and make HIV testing and counselling readily available to a patient with symptoms that may be HIV-related may have an adverse impact on treatment outcomes.[60,61]

It is recommended that TB suspects, defined as any person being evaluated for tuberculosis (through clinical evaluation, smear microscopy or chest radiography), in addition to TB patients, should be tested for HIV infection for several reasons. First, TB suspects have signs and symptoms that could indicate HIV infection and therefore meet the criteria outlined above. Second, studies in sub-Saharan Africa have shown that the HIV prevalence rate in TB suspects who are not diagnosed with TB can be the same as, or higher than that of those diagnosed with TB.[62] Finally, HIV status affects the approach to TB diagnosis. Different diagnostic algorithms for TB apply to people living with HIV than to those without HIV infection.[63]

No data on the prevalence of HIV infection among TB suspects in the Western Pacific Region are currently available, however, so it is not possible to assess the potential impact of this activity. In countries with a high HIV prevalence rate among TB patients, such as Cambodia and Papua New Guinea in the Western Pacific Region (and areas of countries with a heterogeneous epidemic, such as

Malaysia and Viet Nam, which have a high prevalence in TB patients), HIV testing should be considered an essential part of the diagnostic evaluation for TB, and thus HIV testing of TB suspects is recommended.[64] Data should be gathered on the prevalence of HIV infection among TB suspects, particularly the burden of HIV among high-risk groups of TB patients, such as injecting drug users.

Special considerations for countries with low HIV prevalence rates in TB patients

In certain countries with a high burden of TB but a very low prevalence of HIV infection in TB patients, such as the Philippines, other options for HIV testing of TB patients may need to be considered. In such settings, scaling-up of testing to meet the needs of TB patients, beyond the general scaling-up of HIV testing services already in process, may not be needed. These countries, along with low prevalence areas of countries with a heterogeneous epidemic, may choose to continue using the referral-based approach to HIV testing, where TB patients are referred to a facility where testing is available and infection-control measures are established. No data are available from countries with a low prevalence of HIV in TB patients to determine which patients should be prioritized for testing.

Scaling up testing

The best practice for all countries for HIV testing of TB patients is to establish provider-initiated testing and counselling at all TB facilities. This is most urgently needed in those countries and subnational geographical areas where HIV prevalence among TB patients is high. However, it is recognized that there are barriers to achieving full coverage of TB patients and TB suspects, and that implementation needs to address those barriers.

The national TB-HIV coordinating body should first match data comparing the location of DOTS clinics to that of actual and planned locations of HIV testing and counselling services. DOTS clinics should be divided into those that are located within the same complex as a testing and counselling site, those located near a testing and counselling site, and those that are more isolated. They should then identify the planned method for PITC at each DOTS clinic. For example, a DOTS clinic that is geographically isolated may need to have TB staff trained to perform counselling, collect blood and perform the test on site, while a DOTS clinic at a large hospital may only need to train staff on counselling and may be able to use the on-site laboratory for HIV testing. For a facility located near an HIV testing facility, the best option may be to carry out counselling and blood collection at the DOTS clinic and transport the blood to the HIV testing facility for laboratory testing. Finally, several low-volume TB facilities located in relatively close geographic proximity may be appropriate sites to implement mobile counselling and testing.

The national TB-HIV coordinating body should then use the available epidemiology to guide scaling-up, which will often take place using a phased approach. The priority sites may be chosen based on many factors, including a high burden of TB cases and suspects, a high HIV prevalence in TB patients, and geographical isolation, such that access to on-site testing is urgently needed.

Once decisions have been made, implementation should follow closely behind. First, staff must be trained in counselling and performance of the laboratory test. As described above, curricula for this have already been developed and used in multiple countries, and the duration of the training required is relatively short. Second, laboratory supervisors are needed for quality control of testing and biosafety supervision at sites. This should not involve a large time commitment. Next, measures for confidentiality should be put in place. In fact, the same confidentiality measures should already be in place for TB services. Confidentiality is also addressed in the training described above. This needs to be addressed in each facility, and it should be part of routine TB programme supervisory activities. Finally, the necessary supplies must be procured.[65]

Further guidance on how to implement HIV testing and counselling with on-site staff is located in Annex 1 of this document and in the WHO publication, *Guidance on provider-initiated testing and counselling in heath facilities*.[66]

6. INTENSIFIED TB CASE-FINDING IN HIV CARE SETTINGS

> **Box 4.** Key points for intensified TB case-finding and isoniazid preventive therapy
>
> - HIV care settings should develop the capacity to screen for and diagnose TB through one of a variety of approaches.
> - All people with HIV should be screened for TB at the time of initial HIV diagnosis, and regularly thereafter.
> - A clinical algorithm can be used to screen for TB. If none of the listed symptoms are present, then the likelihood of TB is very small and further screening is generally not needed.
> - When TB is ruled out through screening, IPT can be started, where it is available.
> - Countries should work to develop an evidence base about the use of IPT in the Western Pacific Region.
> - Countries should work to scale up use of liquid culture to improve the diagnosis of TB in people with HIV.

The prevalence of latent TB infection is high throughout the Western Pacific Region.[67] Because of this, people living with HIV in countries in the Region are at high risk for TB disease. Where studied, the prevalence of TB disease in patients newly diagnosed with HIV infection is as high as 25%.[68] While the implementation of HIV testing of TB patients may vary across countries in the Western Pacific Region due to the differing HIV prevalence rates, the high prevalence of latent TB infection and high TB incidence rates throughout the Region make rapid countrywide scaling-up of intensified TB case-finding essential for all countries.

Since people with both TB and HIV have very high early case-fatality rates, identifying TB early in an HIV-infected person is very important. Likewise, accurately diagnosing and treating TB increases the safety of ART initiation, while excluding TB identifies patients who may benefit from IPT. The emphasis of intensified case finding should not be only on the diagnosis of smear-positive disease, but rather on early detection of all forms of TB, since all forms of TB in people living with HIV result in increased case-fatality rates and also preclude the use of IPT. Given the high burden of TB throughout the Region, TB screening is considered very important in the HIV programmes of all countries.

There are barriers to TB diagnosis that must be overcome. These include: (1) stigma and perceived stigma, among both health care workers and patients; (2) the cost of TB treatment and diagnosis in countries in which these are not available free of charge; and (3) a lack of knowledge about the risk of TB or an inaccurate perception of the risk.[69]

Approach to TB screening and diagnosis

Where should TB screening and diagnosis take place?

If strong referral systems are in place from HIV testing facilities to HIV treatment facilities, such that there is little delay prior to presentation at the HIV treatment facility, then TB screening can be done at the HIV treatment facility. Where such referral systems are not as strong or delays are common, then TB screening must be made available within HIV testing facilities to avoid delays in TB diagnosis, which could ultimately cost lives.

Since TB is the most common and most deadly OI among people living with HIV in the Region, the capacity to accurately screen for and diagnose TB should exist or be created within all HIV treatment facilities and any diagnostic facility in which TB screening is deemed a necessary activity. This approach is preferred over the routine practice of referring people living with HIV to TB care facilities, as this referral process results in the unnecessary exposure of people living with HIV to TB, which places them at risk of infection and creates unnecessary delays. It is understood that, for certain complicated or challenging cases, referral may be needed. In general, however, HIV care and treatment facilities should have the capacity to do a symptom screen for all patients, obtain and read a chest radiograph when necessary, and obtain sputum specimens for smear microscopy (this can be done by sending the patient to a laboratory or by collecting the sputum and sending that to the TB diagnostic laboratory). Potential approaches to diagnosis of TB in HIV care settings include: (1) placing a TB staff member in the HIV care setting to evaluate patients for TB; (2) training HIV staff to screen for and diagnose TB; or (3) integrating TB and HIV care as part of the decentralization of care.

Who should be screened?

All people living with HIV should be screened for TB disease at diagnosis, prior to starting ART, and at regular intervals thereafter.[70] The times at which TB is most commonly found are at initial HIV diagnosis, during the period prior to ART initiation, and shortly after ART initiation.[71,72]

What screening should be done?

Published data on the best approach to TB screening among people living with HIV are very limited. The prevalence of TB at initial HIV diagnosis can be very high.[73] This is also the time when TB diagnosis is the most challenging, as patients are often very immunosuppressed.[74,75,76] Such patients more commonly have negative sputum smears,[77] normal chest radiographs,[78] and fewer typical TB symptoms than their immunocompetent counterparts.[79,80] For this reason, the appropriate approach to screening may be different for patients at initial presentation than for routine follow-up. More sensitive testing may be warranted at initial presentation, although data are not yet available to confirm this.

A recent WHO publication, *Improving the diagnosis of smear-negative and extrapulmonary tuberculosis among adults and adolescents*,[81] outlines an algorithm for diagnosing TB among people living with HIV in an ambulatory setting. However, this algorithm only applies to the diagnostic evaluation of persons who have a cough. Data from the Western Pacific Region suggest that different criteria may be needed for people with both TB and HIV to enter into this algorithm. In Cambodia, one study found that a cough >3 weeks was only 55% sensitive and 59% specific for a culture-confirmed diagnosis of TB.[82] This study found that a symptom complex of rapid weight loss (over weeks to months, as self-reported by the patient), fever and haemoptysis (where screening was counted as positive for patients with at least one of those symptoms) was 100% sensitive for the diagnosis. Preliminary data from a second study in Cambodia, Thailand and Viet Nam found that a cough >3 weeks was just 21% sensitive, and a cough >2 weeks just 25% sensitive for a culture-confirmed diagnosis of TB. When any one of: cough, self-reported fever or self-reported weight-loss were used, the sensitivity was >90%.[83] The negative predictive value of this screening approach is >97%, thus a patient who has none of the three symptoms is very unlikely to have TB. Recent data from Ethiopia found that a cough of any duration was just 44% sensitive for culture-confirmed TB diagnosis, but that the combination of weight-loss, fever and cough was 86% sensitive.[84] It is clear from the available data that a cough >2 or 3 weeks is insufficiently sensitive to use alone for screening. However, more data are urgently needed to determine the best algorithm for TB screening and diagnosis among people living with HIV. In the interim, however, the algorithm included in the above-mentioned WHO document has been adapted using these additional data, thus using as the entry point any patient with weight loss, fever or a cough (Figure 2). Countries in the Region may choose to further adapt this algorithm based on their local situations.

The use of this algorithm is recommended for all people living with HIV at diagnosis and at regular intervals prior to starting ART.[85] After starting ART, it is possible less sensitive criteria for entry to the algorithm, including those outlined in the WHO document, could be used. However, data are currently insufficient to make this determination and thus it is recommended that the algorithms shown in this document be used whenever screening is done. A separate algorithm for seriously ill patients is available in the WHO publication, *Improving the diagnosis of smear-negative and extrapulmonary tuberculosis among adults and adolescents*.[86] This may be used for TB diagnosis among seriously ill people living with HIV in the Western Pacific Region, except that the entry criteria for the algorithm should be modified to include any patient with a cough, fever or weight loss.

No internationally accepted, evidence-based approaches to screening for extrapulmonary TB yet exist. The WHO document referenced above proposes some criteria that may help with the diagnosis, but data are not currently available to guide the approach.

When to screen for TB

TB screening using the algorithm provided should be done at diagnosis and at every follow-up visit.[87]

TB treatment

Any patient diagnosed with tuberculosis according to this algorithm should immediately be registered for TB treatment and placed on appropriate therapy, in accordance with national policy. Depending on the health facility, treatment may be provided at the HIV treatment facility (if DOTS is available there) or at a location convenient for the patient.

Drug-resistant tuberculosis

Multidrug-resistant (MDR) tuberculosis is TB that is resistant to both isoniazid and rifampicin. Extensively drug-resistant (XDR) TB is MDR TB with additional resistance to two categories of second-line TB drugs, fluoroquinolones and the injectibles, amikacin or kanamycin.[88,89] people living with HIV who develop MDR or XDR TB are at very high risk for early death. In South Africa, 53 people living with HIV with XDR TB were reported in one region of the country, and 52 of them died. The median time from diagnosis to death was just 16 days.[90]

WHO recommends that surveillance for TB drug resistance is carried out at regular intervals.[91] Such surveillance should help countries to determine which patients need culture and drug-susceptibility testing, and countries should develop guidelines on this. In some countries, it may include all re-treatment patients. When needed, such testing should be done as early as possible, as the early case-fatality rate is very high.

Tuberculosis laboratory issues

The diagnosis of tuberculosis in people living with HIV is more difficult than in persons without HIV infection. It is thus essential that high-quality laboratory services are available for people with both TB and HIV. Quality-assured smear microscopy should be available for TB screening for all people living with HIV.

However, even with high-quality smear microscopy, many cases of TB will still be missed, and smear microscopy cannot detect drug resistance. Liquid culture is currently the most sensitive and fastest method available for TB diagnosis. It also allows for drug-susceptibility testing. Liquid culture is the 'gold standard' of care for TB diagnosis, but currently its availability in most resource-limited settings is limited. However, its feasibility and impact have been demonstrated in the Philippines and Thailand, and scaling-up of its use is ongoing in several sub-Saharan African countries.[92]

It is recommended that countries work to scale up access to liquid culture.[93] For some, this may mean implementing liquid culture in a small number of places (or even just one national location) and developing transportation networks to send specimens to the laboratories for culture, as needed. However, efforts to integrate the more routine use of TB culture into TB screening for people living with HIV are needed, and countries are encouraged to develop plans specific to their situations. Plans to scale up liquid culture should generally be part of a comprehensive laboratory-strengthening plan.

Prevention of tuberculosis: isoniazid preventive therapy

For patients in whom tuberculosis is excluded based on the guidance above, IPT may be warranted. IPT involves a six-month course of daily isoniazid, which is given to people living with HIV with latent TB infection in order to prevent the development of active TB disease.[94] IPT has been shown to decrease TB incidence among people living with HIV with latent TB infection by up to 60%, although studies have not yet demonstrated that it improves survival and the duration of protection is limited.[95,96,97,98]

HIV-infected persons are eligible for IPT if they either have none of the symptoms listed above, which would prompt further TB evaluation (weight loss, fever or a cough), or they do have one or more of these symptoms but their chest radiograph is not consistent with TB, they are not diagnosed with extrapulmonary TB by their provider, and their sputum culture is negative. Some countries may choose to use more stringent screening techniques. However, at a minimum, the patient should be evaluated for a combination of symptoms, as described. In multiple randomized controlled clinical trials in high-burden TB countries, the benefit of IPT has been limited to patients with a positive tuberculin skin test (TST) result. However, in many countries, the use of TST is a major challenge. In countries that do not wish to use TST, or find it is not feasible, IPT can be started without TST. For countries that prefer to use TST, this approach is acceptable as well. While TST is useful, it is not necessary for an IPT programme to use it.[99] For more details on other considerations regarding IPT, please see the WHO *TB-HIV clinical manual*.[100] It should be noted that the algorithms presented in this document are those recommended for TB screening and diagnosis in the Western Pacific Region and differ from those listed in the clinical manual.

Isoniazid, as with other TB drugs and antiretroviral drugs, does have side-effects, and patients receiving IPT should be monitored for the development of hepatotoxicity.[101] Such monitoring is especially important for persons with hepatitis B or C. These conditions are not contraindications for isoniazid, but they do necessitate closer monitoring.

FIGURE 2. Algorithm for TB screening for ambulatory people living with HIV

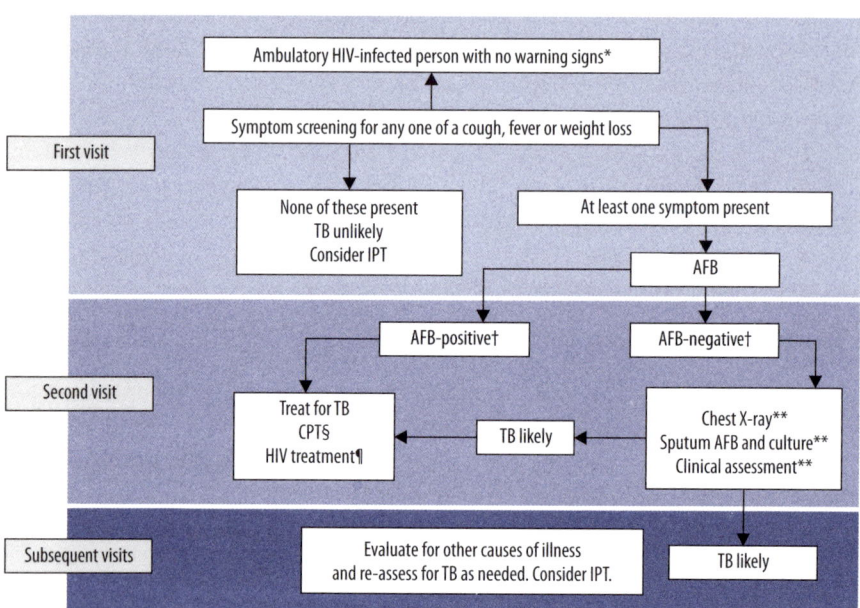

* Warning signs include any one of: respiratory rate >30/minute, fever >39 °C, pulse rate >120/min and unable to walk unaided.
† AFB-positive is defined as at least one positive smear and AFB-negative as two or more negative smears.
§ CPT = Co-trimoxazole preventive therapy. Administer as per national guidelines.
¶ HIV treatment includes CD4 and clinical staging, as well as referral for HIV treatment.
** The investigations within the box should be done at the same time wherever possible in order to decrease the number of visits and speed up diagnosis. If culture is not available, then the decision should be made based on chest X-ray and clinical assessment, as per national guidelines.

Source: modified from: *Improving the diagnosis and treatment of smear-negative pulmonary and extrapulmonary tuberculosis among adults and adolescents: recommendations for HIV-prevalent and resource-constrained settings.* Geneva, World Health Organization, 2007.

7. TREATMENT FOR PEOPLE WITH BOTH TB AND HIV

HIV-infected TB patients in the Western Pacific Region have a very high early case-fatality rate. If only TB treatment is provided, up to 25%-56% will die within 6-12 months of diagnosis.[102,103,104,105] Detecting TB-HIV co-infection early is a critical first step. Providing appropriate treatment early, using antituberculosis therapy along with antiretroviral therapy and prophylaxis for opportunistic infections, is the only way to decrease the risk of death for co-infected people.

This section outlines some treatment considerations for people with both TB and HIV in the Western Pacific Region. Further guidance can be found in the WHO *TB-HIV clinical manual.*[106]

Antituberculosis therapy

HIV-infected TB patients should be registered and started immediately on standard antituberculosis therapy. No modifications to the standard antituberculosis regimens are currently recommended for people living with HIV.

Antiretroviral therapy

More details about the use of ART can be found in the WHO publication, *Antiretroviral therapy for HIV infection in adults and adolescents: recommendations for a public health approach.*[107] This document devotes an entire section to the use of ART in people with both TB and HIV.

Rationale

Antiretroviral therapy clearly decreases the risk of death among people with both TB and HIV. In Ubon Ratchathani, Thailand, 43% of people with both TB and HIV who were not treated with ART died during TB treatment, compared with 7% of people with both TB and HIV who did receive ART.[108] Likewise, an infectious diseases referral hospital near Bangkok reports a one-year case-fatality rate of 56% for people with both TB and HIV without ART, and 4% with ART.[109] In Cambodia, the case-fatality rate for people with both TB and HIV who were treated with ART was 10% after one to two years of follow-up, exactly the same as that for people living with HIV without TB who received ART.[110] Thus, it is clear that prompt diagnosis and treatment of TB-HIV co-infection saves lives.

Who should receive antiretroviral therapy?

According to WHO guidance, all people living with HIV with extrapulmonary TB are eligible for ART, regardless of CD4 count, and people living with HIV with pulmonary TB are eligible for ART if their CD4 count is <350.[111] Eligibility criteria vary by country. However, since most people with both TB and HIV in the Western Pacific Region are very immunosuppressed at the time of diagnosis, almost all of them will qualify immediately for ART, even when more restrictive CD4 criteria are in place, and therefore clinicians should evaluate the eligibility for ART in HIV-infected TB patients promptly.[112,113,114,115]

When to start ART

The most appropriate timing for ART initiation in people with both TB and HIV is controversial and the subject of several ongoing research projects. Observational data from the infectious disease referral centre near Bangkok, Thailand, clearly demonstrate a survival benefit for patients initiating ART within six months of diagnosis of TB-HIV co-infection compared with those starting later (case-fatality of 4.1% in the former group compared with 11.3% in the latter). There was a trend toward decreased case-fatality for people with both TB and HIV starting ART<2 months after diagnosis, in whom the case-fatality rate was 4.2%, compared with the 8.2% case-fatality rate in those starting after two months.[116]

The high early case-fatality rate of people with both TB and HIV and the demonstrated benefit of ART suggest that earlier treatment is the best choice. However, the risk of immune reconstitution inflammatory syndrome may be higher with earlier ART initiation. Current WHO guidelines suggest that, in people with both TB and HIV with CD4<200, ART should be initiated after two weeks of TB treatment, and after the patient is stabilized on the TB regimen. In people with both TB and HIV with CD4 of 200-350, ART should be started after eight weeks of TB therapy, and in people with both TB and HIV with CD4>350, ART can be deferred until after TB therapy is complete.[117]

These guidelines may change at any time, since this topic is currently under careful investigation. This approach is appropriate until further research is completed that demonstrates the most appropriate time to initiate therapy, or the WHO guidelines, *Antiretroviral therapy for HIV infection in adults and adolescents: recommendations for a public health approach*,[118] are updated.

ART regimen

There are important drug-drug interactions between rifampicin, which is typically included in TB regimens throughout the Region, and certain antiretroviral drugs, including nevirapine, which is a commonly used first-line antiretroviral drug. Normally, an alternative antiretroviral agent, such as efavirenz, is substituted for nevirapine during the time that the patient is taking rifampicin. However, efavirenz is contraindicated in pregnancy. For details about selecting an ART regimen for people with both TB and HIV, please consult the WHO publication, *Antiretroviral therapy for HIV infection in adults and adolescents: recommendations for a public health approach*.[119,120]

Treatment adherence

Both TB and HIV treatment require long-term therapy with multiple medications, and adherence is an essential aspect of successful treatment. Efforts should be made to support adherence through means that may include appropriate education and counselling, nutritional support and community-based support.

Adverse effects

HIV-infected TB patients who are treated with antiretroviral therapy are subject to the usual array of adverse effects from such therapy. However, a special concern for people with both TB and HIV who start ART is immune reconstitution inflammatory syndrome (IRIS). This syndrome is a paradoxical worsening of clinical disease after initial improvement. It may occur in up to one-third of TB patients who start ART, and it typically occurs within three months of ART initiation. In severe cases, it can cause death. Corticosteroids are sometimes used to treat severe cases. More complete information about this and other adverse effects are available in the document, *Antiretroviral therapy for HIV infection in adults and adolescents: recommendations for a public health approach*.[121]

Prophylaxis for opportunistic infections

Because they are very immunosuppressed at diagnosis, people with both TB and HIV in the Western Pacific Region are susceptible to a wide range of opportunistic infections (OI). Appropriate prophylaxis to prevent these OI may improve survival. Worldwide, CPT is recommended for all people with both TB and HIV. In several studies in sub-Saharan Africa, it improved survival in people with both TB and HIV compared with a placebo. Its benefit is typically ascribed to decreasing the incidence of malaria, PCP and a variety of bacterial infections.[122,123,124,125,126] The epidemiology of OI is different in the Western Pacific Region, however, from that in sub-Saharan Africa, thus the most appropriate prophylaxis regimens may also differ.

A cross-sectional survey of OI among hospitalized people living with HIV in Ho Chi Minh City, Viet Nam, reported that, among 100 people living with HIV, 37% had TB, 34% had wasting syndrome, 16% had fungal infections (9% with cryptococcosis, 7% with penicilliosis), and 5% had PCP.[127] A similar survey in Cambodia found that 41% of hospitalized people living with HIV had diarrhoea, 26% had TB, 13% had cryptococcal meningitis, 8% had PCP and 5% had meningitis.[128] A blood-culture survey of febrile people living with HIV in Bangkok, Thailand, found mycobacteremia in 31% and fungemia in 21%.[129] Observational data from Thailand found no association between CPT use and death,[130,131] but one study did find that the risk of death was lower among people with both TB and HIV prescribed fluconazole after diagnosis, compared with those not receiving fluconazole.[132] These findings may be due to the higher burden of fungal disease among patients in this Region compared with sub-Saharan Africa and to the much lower burden of malaria and relatively lower burden of other bacterial diseases in this Region compared with others. One observational study in Viet Nam did demonstrate a significant improvement in survival among people with both TB and HIV treated with CPT.[133]

While the benefit of CPT in the Western Pacific Region is not as clear as it is in sub-Saharan Africa, since it has a strong positive effect on survival in other parts of the world and the data in Asia are insufficient to separately analyse its benefit here, it should be used for all people with both TB and HIV.

The relatively high burden of fungal disease in studies in the Region and in Thailand, along with the survival benefit of fluconazole seen in observational data, suggest that fluconazole may be appropriate OI prophylaxis for people with both TB and HIV. This is consistent with the profound immunosuppression seen among TB-HIV co-infected patients in the Region. Further study is needed regarding the benefit of fluconazole prophylaxis, but its use could be considered.

All people with both TB and HIV are eligible for co-trimoxazole preventive therapy, regardless of CD4 count. CPT may be given by TB facilities or HIV care facilities. The goal should be to ensure that people with both TB and HIV begin taking CPT on the day that they are diagnosed with TB-HIV co-infection if they are not on it already.

8. TB INFECTION CONTROL

HIV-infected persons are highly susceptible to infection with TB and development of TB disease.[134] Since TB is the most common opportunistic infection in people living with HIV, it is common for TB patients, whether diagnosed or undiagnosed, to be present in HIV care settings. To address this, WHO developed a document entitled *Tuberculosis infection control in the era of expanding HIV care and treatment*.[135] This document describes a comprehensive approach to infection control in HIV care settings and should be used to develop and implement appropriate infection-control plans and procedures in all HIV care settings throughout the Western Pacific Region, including client-initiated HIV testing centres, HIV treatment facilities, sites for PLWHA support-group meetings, and certain 'closed settings', including prisons and drug treatment and rehabilitation centres.

All countries should implement a 'minimum package' of infection control activities, which should be scaled up rapidly throughout the country. These should include: (1) development of a national TB infection control framework or guideline; (2) training of health care workers on infection control policies; (3) placement of written guidelines within all TB and HIV care facilities; (4) ensuring good ventilation within all facilities in which TB patients are present; (5) ensuring an adequate supply of face masks for patients to use to practice 'cough etiquette'; and (6) establishing a good system for monitoring and evaluation, including what indicators should be collected and who should supervise the activities. In addition, infection control measures should address the risks of TB in staff of health care facilities. Free TB screening should be available to all staff (including health care workers and other clinic staff). Staff should also have ready access to HIV testing; assignment to areas that do not involve contact with TB patients should be considered for HIV-infected staff.

The most effective measures for infection control are administrative, or workplace, control measures, thus this should be the highest priority for implementation. Administrative, or workplace, control measures refer to approaches that prevent droplet nuclei containing *Mycobacterium tuberculosis* from being generated in a facility. While routine referral of TB patients from TB clinics to HIV care settings for diagnosis, and vice-versa, is largely avoided by approaches recommended in this framework, TB patients will still be in HIV care settings for HIV treatment. Diagnosing TB and initiating appropriate treatment as early as possible, as described in the section in this document on intensified TB case finding, is one effective measure to decrease TB transmission in people living with HIV. A second effective approach is to separate patients with TB from those without. This can be done by separating people living with HIV from TB patients and decreasing the amount of time that TB patients and suspects are in HIV care facilities.[136] In addition to the approaches outlined in the above guidelines, several steps within the context of this framework can be taken to reduce the exposure of people living with HIV o TB patients. These are described below and summarized in Box 5.

> **Box 5.** Key administrative measures to decrease the transmission of tuberculosis to people living with HIV within the context of the regional TB-HIV framework
>
> - Diagnose and treat TB as early as possible through intensified case-finding.
> - Minimize referral of people living with HIV to TB clinics or TB wards for TB screening. These referrals unnecessarily expose people living with HIV to TB. Instead, provide on-site TB screening and diagnosis at HIV care facilities.
> - Minimize referral of TB patients to client-initiated counselling and testing facilities. These referrals unnecessarily expose people living with HIV at these testing sites to TB. Instead, implement on-site HIV testing at TB clinics.
> - Establish mechanisms to provide ART at the few specialized TB facilities that provide treatment for MDR and XDR TB. By providing ART on site, HIV-infected MDR and XDR TB patients get the care they need without exposing people living with HIV at HIV care facilities to drug-resistant TB.
> - In facilities where people living with HIV are present, separate suspected or known TB patients and coughing patients from other people living with HIV.
> - Encourage 'cough etiquette'; provide patients with surgical masks or some other barrier to use when coughing.
> - Sputum collection should be done outside or in a well-ventilated area specifically designed for that purpose.

HIV testing of TB patients should be done on site in TB facilities. HIV testing facilities commonly have many people living with HIV present, whether diagnosed or undiagnosed. Sending TB patients to HIV testing facilities needlessly exposes people living with HIV to infectious TB. As documented previously, on-site HIV testing is feasible even in the smallest, most rural health facilities, as no electricity, running water or formal laboratory is needed and the testing does not require a laboratory technician.[137]

Similarly, people living with HIV should not be routinely sent to a TB clinic or TB ward for TB screening, but rather should be screened on site in the HIV care facility, in order to avoid unnecessary exposure to infectious TB patients. This can be accomplished by ensuring that HIV providers are adequately trained to diagnose TB or by having a TB provider work in the HIV care facility.

Antiretroviral therapy is typically not available at TB clinics, although it has been successfully implemented in some TB clinics worldwide. As demonstrated earlier, ART is an essential component of TB-HIV treatment. However, sending people with both TB and HIV to the HIV treatment facility for care exposes other people living with HIV there to tuberculosis. At times, this may not be entirely avoidable, and HIV care and treatment facilities should prepare for this and implement appropriate infection-control procedures. These procedures should include at a minimum: (1) separating patients with smear-positive pulmonary TB from other people living with HIV; (2) separating patients with a cough from those without a cough; (3) encouraging 'cough etiquette', including providing patients with surgical masks or other barriers for their cough; and (4) ensuring that sputum collection is done outside or in a well-ventilated area specifically designed for that purpose.

It is strongly recommended that the few specialized TB facilities that treat MDR TB also develop the capacity to provide ART. Patients with MDR TB are infectious for a much longer period than patients with drug-sensitive TB, and transmission of MDR TB to people living with HIV commonly results in death. Since the consequences of transmission are substantial, training staff at such facilities to provide ART, or having an HIV provider work at such a facility at regular intervals, is strongly recommended.

9. TB-HIV CO-INFECTION IN CHILDREN

TB-HIV co-infection is an important issue in children, as it is in adults, and the recommendations provided in this framework should not be limited to adults, but should also extend to the management of children. All children with TB (and those suspected of having TB) should be tested for HIV infection. HIV testing should ideally be available on site at the facility where TB treatment is provided and should be done using the PITC approach. All children with HIV should be screened for TB at initial HIV diagnosis and regularly thereafter. Children without TB should be considered for IPT, where such treatment is available, and persons with both TB and HIV should be treated appropriately for both diseases, including having early access to ART. [138]

Addressing TB and HIV in children does, however, require addressing certain challenges not encountered in the adult population, particularly in the areas of TB screening and diagnosis in children with HIV, and the use of the BCG vaccine.

Diagnosing TB can be more challenging in children than in adults. This is largely due to the difficulty in obtaining sputum from a young child and often requires the use of additional techniques, such as gastric aspiration or sputum induction. While TB diagnosis in children typically requires evaluation by health care staff with skill and experience in this area, all health care staff who care for people with HIV should be trained to recognize the signs and symptoms of TB in children.[139]

Children who are contacts of TB cases are at high risk for TB disease and should be evaluated for TB infection. Where TST and chest radiography are not readily available, clinical assessment should be used to identify children requiring further evaluation for TB disease and those who should receive IPT. Household contact investigations are useful to detect TB in children who live with a person who has been diagnosed with TB.[140]

Finally, BCG vaccination is contraindicated in persons with impaired immunity, and WHO does not recommend BCG vaccination in children with symptomatic HIV infection. It is recognized that some programmes may lack the ability to accurately diagnose HIV in an infant whose mother is infected with HIV. This situation is addressed in detail in articles in the *Weekly epidemiological record*.[141,142]

10. MONITORING AND EVALUATION

Collecting high quality data and tracking appropriate monitoring and evaluation indicators is important for ongoing programme improvement. Responsibilities for recording, reporting, monitoring and evaluation need to be clearly stated between TB and HIV programmes. In addition, information systems for TB and HIV need to be rapidly upgraded to capture essential TB-HIV co-infection information.

WHO has published several monitoring and evaluation indicators in the document, *A guide to monitoring and evaluation for collaborative TB-HIV activities*, along with additional indicators in the *Monitoring and evaluation toolkit*.[143,144] The indicators which should be used for monitoring and evaluation of activities outlined in this regional framework are listed in Boxes 6, 7, and 8. These indicators can be used for monitoring and evaluation at the national, subnational and facility level, and countries should develop appropriate targets for eah of them.

> **Box 6.** Core indicators for monitoring collaborative TB-HIV activities in the Western Pacific Region
>
> 1. Proportion of individuals newly enrolled in HIV care starting isoniazid preventive therapy (IPT).
> 2. Percentage of TB patients who have had an HIV test result recorded in the TB register (also include number and percentage who are HIV-positive).
> 3. Percentage of newly registered HIV-infected TB patients started on or continuing co-trimoxazole preventive therapy (CPT).
> 4. Percentage of people with both TB and HIV who were started on ART or continued previously initiated ART, during or at the end of TB treatment.
>
> Sources: [1] *Guide to monitoring and evaluation for collaborative TB/HIV activities.* Geneva, World Health Organization 2004. [2] *Monitoring and evaluation toolkit: HIV/AIDS, tuberculosis and malaria.* 2nd ed. Geneva, Global Fund to Fight AIDA, Tuberculosis and Malaria, 2006.

Collecting, monitoring and evaluating data for TB screening and diagnosis among people living with HIV is a challenge. When collecting data on screening during follow-up visits, it is difficult to establish a useful denominator. However, ensuring that patients are screened regularly is important. Thus, the core indicators for measuring TB screening and diagnosis in people living with HIV have been modified slightly. These indicators separately collect data on TB screening at initial HIV diagnosis, at which time TB is most common and where the denominator is easily established, and TB screening during follow-up. These modified indicators are shown in Box 7.

> **Box 7.** Modified core indicators for TB screening in people living with HIV
>
> 5. Percentage of HIV-infected patients screened for tuberculosis according to the algorithm provided at initial HIV diagnosis (also include the number diagnosed with TB and registered for TB treatment).*
>
> 6. Percentage of people living with HIV (on ART and not yet on ART) screened for TB at the most recent visit (also include the number diagnosed with TB and registered for TB treatment).*
>
> * These indicators have been modified slightly compared with those in: [1] *Guide to monitoring and evaluation for collaborative TB/HIV activities.* Geneva, World Health Organization 2004. [2] *Monitoring and evaluation toolkit: HIV/AIDS, tuberculosis and malaria.* 2nd ed. Geneva, Global Fund to Fight AIDA, Tuberculosis and Malaria, 2006.

Finally, since a key aspect of this framework is to implement TB-HIV activities that are, not only appropriate for ensuring early diagnosis and treatment, but also for serving as administrative controls (methods of decreasing the exposure of people living with HIV to infectious TB patients) in a broader infection control plan, the indicators in Box 8 are used to capture data on this progress.

> **Box 8.** Indicators which capture progress on key aspects of this framework
>
> 7. The number of TB facilities offering PITC (defined as HIV testing that does not require the patient to go to a client-initiated testing facility or VCT site), expressed as a proportion of all TB facilities in the country.*
>
> 8. The number of hub HIV treatment facilities offering on-site TB screening and diagnosis, expressed as a proportion of the total number of hub HIV treatment facilities in the country.*
>
> 9. The number of MDR TB treatment facilities providing ART on site, expressed as a proportion of all facilities that provide MDR TB treatment in the country.*
>
> 10. Infection control: Age and sex-adjusted TB notification rate ratio in health care staff compared with the general population ≤1.
>
> 11. Case-fatality rate of HIV-infected TB patients, calculated as a proportion of newly registered TB patients who are HIV-infected, whose TB treatment outcome is "died".
>
> 12. TB incidence in HIV patients.
>
> *These are indicators specifically designed for this framework.

11. TB-HIV IN 'CLOSED SETTINGS' AND AMONG INJECTING DRUG USERS

Special consideration is needed to address TB-HIV co-infection in 'closed settings', which include, but are not limited to: drug and alcohol treatment or rehabilitation centres, forced (or compulsory) treatment centres and prisons. In many countries the TB and HIV incidence rates are extremely high in confined populations,[145] both higher than in the community (sometimes 10-50 times higher). Additionally, prisons and other forms of closed setting are normally facilities where access to basic health care is more often neglected and where commitments to improve the health condition of the incarcerated are not commonly established. Furthermore, closed settings are usually associated with coercion and forced initiatives 'to promote health', with a clear lack of negotiation capability or preservation of the basic rights that the same person can have in the community.

These settings should offer HIV testing and TB screening as outlined previously. It is essential that HIV testing should never be mandatory or coerced. Systems for maintaining confidentiality should be clearly established in these settings. Countries are encouraged to review relevant laws to ensure that they are consistent with easy access to voluntary and confidential HIV testing, TB screening and TB-HIV care. Provider-initiated testing and counselling is an appropriate approach to HIV testing within such populations. More details about implementing PITC are found in section 5 and Annex 1 of this document, and in the WHO document *Guidance on provider-initiated testing and counselling in health facilities*.[146]

It is crucial to establish treatment programmes or a clear referral system for tuberculosis and HIV in closed settings. After screening for TB and HIV, patients diagnosed with either or both diseases should be treated using the same standards as would apply in the community. Attention must also be given to referral to community services in cases of release from a closed setting or referral from such services for admission to a closed setting. In some countries, NGOs play a very important role in the linking the prison system and the public health system in order to support the continuity of treatment for both diseases, which is a key element in enhancing treatment adherence.

Finally, because HIV infection and TB are common in these settings, the same infection control guidelines outlined in the document, *Tuberculosis infection control in the era of expanding HIV care and treatment*, should also be applied in these settings.[147] This includes having facilities to provide treatment to TB patients in an area that is separated from other persons. Special attention should be given to MDR TB, since it has been proven that closed settings are among the highest-risk places for its development.[148] Training in TB and HIV is desirable for health staff working for the prison system.

People who inject drugs

In many communities throughout the world, the HIV/AIDS, TB and substance abuse epidemics are intertwined, each contributing to the increased incidence, morbidity and mortality of the other. Injecting drug use is a leading mode of HIV transmission and accounts for 30% of the global burden of the disease outside Sub-Saharan Africa.[149] This mode of transmission is particularly important in Asia and the Western Pacific Region. People who inject drugs are a population at high risk for both TB and HIV. Among people living with HIV who also inject drugs, TB is a leading cause of mortality.

Due to the high level of criminalization attached to drug-usage behaviour in the majority of countries in the Western Pacific Region, many people who inject drugs have also experienced (or will experience) incarceration in the form of prison or compulsory treatment. Providing early access to TB and HIV diagnosis and treatment for this segment of the population is very important. It is important to provide training on TB and HIV for outreach workers and drug-dependence treatment staff. Needle and syringe programmes, methadone clinics and other facilities dedicated to people who inject drugs can be the target for such training sessions. The linkage of prevention strategies and the control of TB among people who inject drugs is being well documented and it is a promising way of confronting co-infection.[150,151]

It is important to note the misconception in the health sector that people who inject drugs do not adhere to long-term treatment. This misconception is also present among health professionals dedicated to the care of confined people. However, evidence suggests that people who inject drugs are as likely to adhere to TB or HIV treatment as other patients.[152,153] People providing services must be trained to deal with this population in a non-judgmental way to improve the chances of success.

Patients on opioid-substitution therapy require special attention due to important interactions between anti-TB drugs and methadone. Rifampicin and the combination of rifampicin and isoniazid cause a substantial decrease in methadone levels (up to 68%), which can induce methadone withdrawal. Using these TB drugs requires careful monitoring and potentially an increase in the methadone dose.[154,155] Some interactions also occur with antiretroviral medications.

WHO (Regional Offices for South-East Asia and the Western Pacific) and UNODC have just produced *HIV/AIDS care and treatment for people who inject drugs in Asia and the Pacific, an essential practice guide,* which may be of help in dealing with drug interactions in the case of HIV treatment and drug treatment or abuse.[156] In addition, new guidelines called *Providing comprehensive TB and HIV prevention, treatment and care services for drug users: an integrated approach* is under preparation by WHO and should be released in 2008, with more detailed recommendations.[157]

12. COMMUNITY LEVEL TB-HIV COLLABORATION

TB and HIV services both exist at the community level and there are important opportunities for collaboration. Two examples of community-based initiatives for TB and HIV are home-based care teams, which typically provide care and services for people living with HIV, and community DOTS programmes, which typically provide TB-related services. Collaboration between these and other community-based programmes can improve TB-HIV control. Through close collaboration with local health facilities, these groups can facilitate early diagnosis of TB and HIV, improve adherence to TB- and HIV-related treatment, and improve treatment outcomes.

Undiagnosed tuberculosis is common among all people living with HIV. A survey of patients in a home-based care programme in Cambodia found that 12% had active TB disease, of which 74% had not been diagnosed previously; 49% of the people with both TB and HIV died within three months of screening.[158] Home-based care services or community DOTS teams could perform symptom screening according to the algorithm provided in this document. Programmes should refer any patient with any one of the three symptoms (weight loss, a cough or fever) to the HIV care facility for further evaluation.

Community-based DOTS programmes can also impact TB-HIV care in other ways. First, they can facilitate TB treatment nearer the patient's home for persons who have difficulty travelling regularly to the health facility. Second, they can assess whether TB patients have been tested for HIV infection. Those who initially declined or were not offered testing can be encouraged to be tested at the TB treatment facility where they are registered for treatment, or at another site of their choice. Finally, community-based DOTS programmes may be able to facilitate TB screening and HIV testing of household contacts of TB patients with and without HIV infection. In a study in Chiang Rai, Thailand, the household contacts of 499 patients with pulmonary TB were screened for TB and tested for HIV infection; 45 contacts were diagnosed with TB disease and 65 with HIV infection (including seven with both TB and HIV).[159] Not only does such screening increase TB case detection and HIV case-finding, it also accomplishes early diagnosis of TB and HIV.

Both community DOTS programmes and home-based care services can work with patients to improve adherence. The long duration of treatment required for both TB and HIV make adherence a challenge, but community-based groups can help to overcome the barriers. Community-based TB-HIV collaboration is important for all patients, but it may be particularly important for drug users and other populations needing special consideration. For such populations, adherence to treatment is high if the right support services are available.

13. PRIORITIES FOR PROGRAMMATICALLY RELEVANT RESEARCH

While, in many cases, the best practices to address TB-HIV are known, there are areas for which optimal care is unknown. Programmatically relevant research into these areas should be carried out in order to improve service delivery and decrease the high case-fatality rates seen in the Region. WHO has developed a document, entitled *TB-HIV research priorities in resource-limited settings*,[160] which outlines important areas in which research is needed. Box 9 highlights some areas which are particularly important research needs n the Western Pacific Region.

Box 9. Priorities for programmatically relevant TB-HIV research in the Western Pacific Region

- Development and validation of algorithms to exclude all forms of TB in people living with HIV.
- Development and validation of algorithms to diagnose smear-negative and extrapulmonary TB in people living with HIV.
- Determination of the most appropriate frequency for TB screening of people living with HIV already in HIV care.
- Assessment of the optimal approach for the delivery of isoniazid preventive therapy.
- Assessment of the impact of co-trimoxazole preventive therapy in the Western Pacific Region, particularly in the context of antiretroviral therapy.
- Assessment of the different strategies for delivery of co-trimoxazole preventive therapy, including possibly giving it along with DOTS drugs.
- Determination of the most appropriate time to start antiretroviral therapy in people with both TB and HIV.
- Assessment of the role of prophylaxis for opportunistic infections caused by fungi and atypical mycobacteria.
- Determination of HIV prevalence in TB suspects in the Western Pacific Region.
- Development of diagnostic algorithms for TB in HIV-infected children.
- Assessment of the impact of new diagnostic techniques as they become available.
- Documentation of the feasibility and impact of implementing liquid culture and other new rapid diagnostic methods in the Region.

ANNEX 1. COUNSELLING AND HIV TESTING USING ON-SITE STAFF

How to do the testing and counselling

Pre-test information

In contrast to the VCT approach, where comprehensive pre-test counselling is performed, with PITC, basic information is provided to patients prior to HIV testing so that they can decide whether or not to accept testing, but a full risk-assessment is not carried out. The rationale for this approach is that patients clearly have an indication for HIV testing. They are not being tested because of their concern about risk, but rather because they have signs or symptoms compatible with HIV infection.[161]

Pre-test information can be provided prior to HIV testing in the form of individual sessions with each patient or in a group, depending on the needs of the health care facility. Informed consent must be given; it can be given verbally and should always be given individually, in private, in the presence of a health care provider.[162] Box 1 outlines the information that should be provided to all patients prior to giving consent

---

Box 1. Minimum pre-test information which should be provided to all patients prior to informed consent being given for HIV testing

- The reasons why HIV testing and counselling is being recommended, namely, that many TB patients and people with symptoms of TB have HIV infection, and that the approach to TB diagnosis and treatment for HIV-infected individuals is different from that for those without HIV infection.

- The clinical and preventive benefits of testing and the potential risks, such as discrimination, abandonment or violence.

- The services that are available in the case of either an HIV-negative or an HIV-positive test result, including whether antiretroviral therapy is available.

- The fact that the test result will be treated confidentially and will not be shared with anyone other than the health care providers directly involved in providing services to the patient.

- The fact that the patient has the right to decline the test and that testing will be performed unless the patient exercises that right.

- The fact that the patient has the right to be referred to a separate HIV testing facility if the patient would prefer to be tested elsewhere.
- The fact that declining an HIV test will not affect the patient's access to services that do not depend upon knowledge of HIV status.
- In the event of an HIV-positive test result, encouragement of disclosure to other persons who may be at risk of exposure to HIV.
- An opportunity to ask the health care provider questions.

Source: Guidance on provider-initiated HIV testing and counselling in health facilities. Geneva, World Health Organization, 2007.

Patients should also be made aware of relevant laws in jurisdictions that mandate the disclosure of HIV status to sexual and/or drug-injecting partners.

Verbal communication is normally adequate for the purpose of obtaining informed consent. Jurisdictions that require written consent are encouraged to review this policy.

Additional information may be warranted for special groups, including pregnant women, children, adolescents and seriously ill patients. Detailed guidance for these cases can be found in the WHO document, *Guidance on provider-initiated testing and counselling in heath facilities.*[163]

Declining an HIV test should not result in reduced quality or denial of services, coercive treatment or breach of confidentiality, nor should it affect a person's access to health services that do not depend on knowledge of HIV status. Individuals declining the test should be offered assistance to access either client-initiated or provider-initiated testing and counselling in the future.[164]

The patient's decision to decline the HIV test should be noted in the medical record so that, at subsequent visits to the health facility, a discussion regarding HIV testing and counselling can be re-initiated.[165]

HIV testing

HIV testing can generally follow one of three approaches: (1) the blood can be drawn and the test done in the DOTS clinic; (2) the blood can be drawn at the DOTS clinic and sent to the on-site laboratory; or (3) the patient can be sent to the on-site laboratory for blood collection and testing. For many tests, a finger stick may replace phlebotomy for blood collection. In facilities that lack a formal laboratory, the first approach will be the only available option. [166]

These approaches have become feasible due to the introduction of sensitive, specific, simple-to-use, rapid antibody tests that do not require sophisticated laboratory services, running water or electricity. Testing can occur outside laboratory settings, does not require specialized equipment, and can be carried out in primary health facilities by appropriately trained non-laboratory personnel, including counsellors and TB staff. Trained laboratory supervisors, however, should provide appropriate supervisory visits to sites implementing PITC for quality assurance, including quality control for testing and bio-safety.[167]

Post-test counselling

Post-test counselling is an integral component of the HIV testing process. All individuals undergoing HIV testing must be counselled when their test results are given, regardless of the test results. Post-test counselling is designed to be brief in the PITC setting, but people living with HIV must all be referred to the HIV treatment facility for full post-test counselling and initiation of care. Given that many inpatient and outpatient facilities are crowded, care should be taken to discuss results and follow-up care in a confidential manner. Results should be given to patients in person by health care providers or by trained lay personnel. Ideally, post-test counselling should be provided by the same health care provider who initiated HIV testing and counselling. Results should not be given in group settings.[168] It is not acceptable for the provider who offered the test to the patient not to know the test result, assuming the patient agreed to be tested. Lack of knowledge of the result on the part of the provider will result in substandard care. Regardless of who provides the test result, the provider should know the result and use it when delivering patient care.

It is likewise not acceptable practice for health care providers to recommend HIV testing and counselling to patients and to subsequently withhold or fail to convey test results. Although patients can refuse to receive or accept results of any tests or investigations, health care providers should make every reasonable attempt to ensure that patients receive their results in a confidential and sympathetic manner and that they understand them.[169] Box 2 shows the recommended components of post-test counselling.

It is recognized that people living with HIV will typically need to be referred for ART, as it is normally not available at TB facilities. Given the high early-mortality rate in people with both TB and HIV, strong mechanisms for referral should be in place such that the patient can access ART as quickly as possible. Alternatively, the provision of ART in TB facilities can be considered. This is the recommended

> **Box 2.** Recommended components of post-test counselling
>
> - Basic prevention services for persons with negative HIV test results:
>   - ◊ Post-test HIV prevention counselling for individuals or couples that includes information about prevention services.
>   - ◊ Promotion and provision of male and female condoms.
>   - ◊ Needle and syringe access and other harm-reduction interventions for injecting drug users.
>   - ◊ Post-exposure prophylaxis, where indicated.
> - Basic services for persons with positive HIV test results:
>   - ◊ Provision of test results in a sensitive manner.
>   - ◊ Immediate referral to HIV care facilities for full post-test counselling and initiation of care.
>   - ◊ Individual post-test counselling by a trained provider that includes information about and referral to prevention, care and treatment services, as required.
>   - ◊ Safer sex and risk-reduction counselling, with promotion and provision of male and female condoms.
>   - ◊ Needle and syringe access and other harm-reduction interventions for injecting drug users.
>
> Source: *Guidance on provider-initiated HIV testing and counselling in health facilities.* Geneva, World Health Organization, 2007.

approach for specialized TB facilities that treat MDR TB, as exposure of people living with HIV to MDR TB must be avoided.

Training

To provide testing and counselling, staff must be trained in counselling techniques and, where needed, laboratory testing techniques. This will often involve training TB staff to provide these services. Training that includes background information, counselling training and laboratory training can be done in a short time. One curriculum that is available on-line provides a four-day training session for this.[170] It was not designed by WHO, and thus there are some differences between it and the WHO approach, but the training can easily be modified to accommodate a country's needs. It was successfully adapted by Thailand and Viet Nam into a three-day training session, which included performing the laboratory test.[171]

Barriers / requirements

As outlined above, there are several essential features required for PITC. First, staff must be trained in counselling and performance of the laboratory test. As described above, curricula for this have already been developed and used in multiple countries, and the duration of the training required is relatively short. Second, laboratory supervisors are needed for quality control of testing and for bio-safety supervision at sites. This should not involve a large time commitment. Finally, measures should be in place to ensure confidentiality. In fact, the same confidentiality measures should already be in place for TB services. Confidentiality is also addressed in the training described above. This needs to be addressed in each facility and should be a part of routine TB programme supervisory activities.

Consideration of each of the above issues is critical. However, given the tremendous benefit of PITC, these should not be considered insurmountable and should not be reasons to avoid it. Instead, addressing these issues should be an important aspect of PITC planning and scaling-up. In many countries, a good approach may be to start with PITC implementation in selected areas, addressing the barriers in the process, and gradually scaling up, as possible.

Other issues, including local laws, stigma and other special considerations. may be important to consider in certain countries. Additional guidance on these issues can be found in the WHO document, *Guidance on provider-initiated testing and counselling in health facilities*.[172]

ANNEX 2. HIV SURVEILLANCE AMONG TB PATIENTS WITH LOW BURDENS OF TB-HIV CO-INFECTION

Motivation

The purpose of surveillance in countries with low burdens of TB-HIV co-infection is to alert authorities when a given level of prevalence has been reached.

Using 2% as an example:

>The null hypothesis to be tested is:
>$H_0: P \geq P_0$ (i.e. the proportion of HIV-infected subjects ≥ 0.02)
>
>The alternative hypothesis is:
>$H_a: P < P_0$ (i.e. the proportion of HIV-infected subjects < 0.02)

The programme manager sets α, the probability of concluding a community has an acceptably low seroprevalence level when it actually has a high level. This type of error (type I) is serious, because the programme manager would decide not to target this community for intervention until the next survey. A type II error, rejection of the null hypothesis when prevalence is actually low, is not so serious.

The hypergeometric distribution is important for representing the probability of observing d infected people in a sample of size n from a population of size N new TB patients, in which NP_0 members are hypothesized to be infected with HIV. The hypergeometric distribution accounts for the fact that the probability of selecting an infected member of the population changes as members are sampled without replacement.

$$P(d \leq d^*) = \sum_{d=0}^{d^*} \frac{\binom{NP_0}{d}\binom{N(1-P_0)}{n-d}}{\binom{N}{n}}$$

If this probability is small relative to α, then it may be concluded that it is unlikely the proportion of HIV-infected new TB patients in the targeted population is as high as P_0. As a result, the TB community would be accepted as a low HIV prevalence area.

The hypergeometric distribution may be used for sample-size determination in the sense that the value of n that is chosen is the one that will yield a hypergeometric probability of less than or equal to α, given the values of P_0, d^* and N stated by the programme manager.

The following table shows sample sizes for n.

TABLE 1. Sample size assuming $\alpha = 0.05$, $P0 = 0.02$

N	$d^* = 0$
500	129
1000	138
2000	143
5000	147
10 000	148
$\geq$50 000	149

Example: if the total number N of new TB patients in a given area during a defined period is 10 000, the null hypothesis that the prevalence of HIV in new TB patients is greater than or equal to 2% cannot be rejected if one or more cases are found infected with HIV out of a sample of 148 tested TB cases. If the sample of 148 tested TB cases yields no HIV-positive test result, then the null hypothesis is rejected and it can be concluded that the prevalence of HIV in the survey area is less than 2%.

Sampling strategy

A sample should be representative of the community it represents. A sampling strategy may involve 30 primary sampling units (PSU), such as hospitals or health centres where TB diagnostic services are available on site, sampled with a probability proportional to size (PPS) from each first-level subnational administrative area, such as a province or region.

TABLE 2. Sampling example

	Province A	Province B
New TB cases the previous year	1500	4200
Sampled clusters (health facilities) [a]	30	30
Design effect [b]	2	2
Sample size* [c]	142	146
Design-adjusted sample size [d = c * b]	284	292
Cluster size [e = d / a]	10	10

* $\alpha = 0.05$, $P_0 = 0.02$

The cluster size should be the sample size (computed according to the outline above), divided by the number of clusters, multiplied by the anticipated design effect and rounded to the next higher integer (e.g. 142 * 2 / 30 = 10 new TB cases per cluster). Consecutive newly diagnosed TB cases may be tested for HIV until the cluster size is reached. The test statistic (number found to be HIV-positive) is then aggregated across PSUs, allowing testing of whether HIV infection in TB cases has reached a certain level (2%) in every first-level subnational administrative area, after adjustment for the sampling design effect. If one or more HIV-infected TB cases is detected in a particular first-level subnational administrative area, then the null hypothesis that HIV-prevalence in TB cases is higher than 2% in that area cannot be rejected.

Software implementation

R is a freely available statistical environment for Windows, Mac OS X and Unix®.[173] The following simple R code can be used to compute sample size under a variety of assumptions:

```
nsize <- function (p0 = 0.02, N = 10000, d = 0, alpha = 0.05)
{
for (n in N:1)
    {
    m = N - n
    k = trunc(p0 * N)
    if (dhyper(d, n, m, k) > alpha)
    break
    }
return(trunc(n)+1)
}
```

The above code can be directly pasted or copied into an R console. It generates a function named *nsize*. In the first example below, the function returns a sample size of *n*=142 under the default assumptions *P0*=0.02, *d*=0 and *N*=10000. In the second example, the returned sample size *n*=258 corresponds to the assumptions *P0*=0.01 and *N*=1000.

```
>
> nsize()
[1] 142
> nsize(p0=0.01, N=1000)
[1] 258
>
```

ANNEX 3. TB DATA FOR COUNTRIES IN THE WESTERN PACIFIC REGION

TABLE 1. TB notification, estimated TB incidence and case-detection rate for all forms of TB and sputum-smear-positives, stratified by country, 2006.

Country	Population (thousands)	TB case notification, 2006			
		All forms		Smear-positive	
		number	rate	number	rate
American Samoa	65	4	6	3	5
Australia	20 530	1159	6	269	1
Brunei Darussalam	382	202	53	128	34
Cambodia	14 197	34 660	244	19 294	136
China	1 320 864	940 889	71	468 291	35
China, Hong Kong	7132	5356	75	1547	22
China, Macao	478	374	78	144	30
Cook Islands	14	1	7	0	0
Fiji	833	114	14	73	9
French Polynesia	259	69	27	24	9
Guam	171	44	26	21	12
Japan	127 953	25 304	20	10 159	8
Kiribati	94	378	404	129	138
Lao People's Democratic Republic	5759	3958	69	3041	53
Malaysia	26 114	16 051	61	9414	36
Marshall Islands	58	138	238	45	78
Micronesia	111	104	94	41	37
Mongolia	2 605	5049	194	2129	82
Nauru	10	12	118	2	20
New Caledonia	238	48	20	9	4
New Zealand	4140	344	8	97	2
Niue	2	0	0	0	0
Northern Mariana Islands	82	51	62	15	18
Palau	20	12	59	6	30
Papua New Guinea	6202	12 620	203	1948	31
Philippines	86 264	147 305	171	85 740	99
Republic of Korea	48 050	37 861	79	11 513	24
Samoa	185	25	13	13	7
Singapore	4382	1314	30	538	12
Solomon Islands	484	371	77	124	26
Tokelau	1	0	0	0	0
Tonga	100	18	18	14	14
Tuvalu	10	9	86	4	38
Vanuatu	221	126	57	42	19
Viet Nam	86 206	97 363	113	56 437	65
Wallis and Futuna	15				
Western Pacific Region	**1 764 231**	**1 331 333**	**75**	**671 254**	**38**

* Estimated rates are calculated by WHO and will appear in the WHO 2008 global tuberculosis control report.
Source: Tuberculosis control in the Western Pacific Region: 2007 report. Manila, WHO Regional Office for the Western Pacific, 2007.

Estimated TB incidence, 2006				Case detection rate		Country
All forms*		Smear-positive*		all new	new ss+	
number	rate	number	rate	%	%	
6	9	3	4	69	115	American Samoa
1329	6	595	3	85	45	Australia
203	53	91	24	94	141	Brunei Darussalam
71 123	501	31 833	224	48	61	Cambodia
1 311 184	99	589 630	45	68	79	China
5182	73	2332	33	99	66	China, Hong Kong
383	80	172	36	95	84	China, Macao
2	16	1	7	47	0	Cook Islands
184	22	83	10	61	88	Fiji
68	26	31	12	98	78	French Polynesia
64	37	29	17	69	73	Guam
35 537	28	15 980	12	69	64	Japan
348	372	157	168	107	82	Kiribati
8827	153	3966	69	43	77	Lao People's Democratic Republic
26 877	103	12 049	46	58	78	Malaysia
127	220	57	99	101	79	Marshall Islands
112	101	50	45	90	82	Micronesia
4920	189	2213	85	97	96	Mongolia
11	106	5	48	112	42	Nauru
55	23	25	10	74	36	New Caledonia
352	9	158	4	95	61	New Zealand
1	43	0	19	0	0	Niue
61	75	28	34	83	54	Northern Mariana Islands
10	51	5	23	116	129	Palau
15 473	250	6898	111	81	28	Papua New Guinea
249 108	289	112 083	130	57	76	Philippines
47 989	100	21, 561	45	74	53	Republic of Korea
36	19	16	9	64	80	Samoa
1128	26	506	12	110	106	Singapore
655	135	295	61	56	42	Solomon Islands
1	56	0	25	0	0	Tokelau
24	25	11	11	74	127	Tonga
31	295	14	133	29	29	Tuvalu
128	58	58	26	98	73	Vanuatu
149 740	174	67 111	78	61	84	Viet Nam
7	46	3	21			Wallis and Futuna
1 931 287	109	868 047	49	66	77	**Western Pacific Region**

ANNEX 4. DETAILS FOR CALCULATION OF INDICATORS

TABLE 1. List of proposed indicators and approach to calculation

No.*	Indicator	Disaggre-gation	Numerator	Denominator	WHO Universal Access Indicator‡	Data source
1	Proportion of individuals newly enrolled in HIV care starting isoniazid preventive therapy (IPT)		Number of individuals newly enrolled in HIV care started on IPT	Number of individuals newly enrolled in HIV care in the last 12 months	# 32	Annual review of facility records/registers documenting individuals newly enrolled in HIV care in the last 12 months (If national policy on INH prophylaxis/ guidelines exist)
2	Percentage of TB patients who have an HIV test result recorded in the TB register	By sero-status	Number of TB patients who have an HIV test result recorded in the TB register *This should include those TB cases that were previously known as HIV-positive or their negative HIV result from previous testing was acceptable to the clinician (e.g. done in the last 3-6 months in a reliable laboratory).*	Total number of TB patients	# 8	National programme records
3	Percentage of newly registered HIV-infected TB who started or continued to receive co-trimoxazole preventive therapy (CPT)		Number of newly registered TB patients recorded as HIV+ who started on or continued to receive CPT	Total number of newly registered TB patients recorded as HIV+	# 31	TB programme records

ANNEX 4 | DETAILS FOR CALCULATION OF INDICATORS   67

No.*	Indicator	Disaggre-gation	Numerator	Denominator	WHO Universal Access Indicator†	Data source
4	Percentage of people with both TB and HIV who started on ART or continued previously initiated ART, during or at the end of TB treatment		Number of adults with HIV infection who are currently receiving antiretroviral therapy in accordance with the nationally approved treatment protocol (or WHO/UNAIDS standards) and who were started on TB treatment (in accordance with national TB programme guidelines) within the reporting year	Number of adults with HIV infection who were reported to have TB during the reporting year	# 30 (modified slightly)	Currently, facility-based ART registers. If reportable, national programme records
5	Percentage of HIV-infected persons screened for tuberculosis according to the algorithm provided at initial HIV diagnosis	By number diagnosed with TB and started on TB treatment	Number of people with HIV documented at their initial visit to have either: (1) none of the symptoms listed in the symptom screen; or (2) one or more of those symptoms present, but underwent further TB diagnostic work-up	Total number of people with HIV newly registered for care (ART or pre-ART)	N/A	National programme records (in many cases, must be enhanced to capture TB screening data)
6	Percentage of people living with HIV (on ART and not yet on ART) screened for TB at the most recent visit	By number diagnosed with TB and started on TB treatment	Number of people with HIV documented at their most recent visit to have either: (1) none of the symptoms listed in the symptom screen; or (2) one or more of those symptoms present, but underwent further TB diagnostic work-up	Number of individual HIV care records examined	# 33	Annual review of facility records or special study
7	Number of TB facilities offering PITC on site, expressed as a proportion of all TB facilities in the country		Number of TB facilities that provide HIV testing to TB patients without referring the patient to a different facility (e.g. a VCT site).	Total number of TB facilities in the country	N/A	TB programme

No.*	Indicator	Disaggregation	Numerator	Denominator	WHO Universal Access Indicator†	Data source
8	Number of hub HIV treatment facilities offering on-site TB screening and diagnosis, expressed as a proportion of the total number of hub HIV treatment facilities in the country		Number of hub HIV treatment facilities that provide TB screening and diagnosis without referral to another facility	Total number of hub HIV treatment facilities in the country	N/A	HIV programme
9	Number of MDR TB treatment facilities that provide antiretroviral therapy on site, expressed as a proportion of all facilities that provide MDR TB treatment in the country		Number of MDR TB treatment facilities that provide antiretroviral therapy on site, without referral to an HIV treatment facility	Total number of facilities providing MDR TB treatment in the country	N/A	TB programme
10	Infection control: ratio of age- and sex-adjusted TB notification rate in health care staff to the general population ≤1		Age- and sex-adjusted TB notification rate among staff of health care facilities	Age- and sex-adjusted TB notification rate in the country	N/A	Currently, special study
11	Case-fatality rate of HIV-infected TB patients, calculated as a proportion of newly registered TB patients who are HIV-infected whose TB treatment outcome is "died".		Number of newly registered TB patients with HIV in a given reporting year whose TB treatment outcome is "died"	Total number of newly registered TB patients with HIV infection in a given reporting year	N/A	TB programme records
12	TB incidence in HIV-infected persons		Number of people with HIV diagnosed with TB in reporting year	Number of people with HIV currently enrolled in care during reporting year	N/A	HIV programme records (likely special study)

*Refers to indicator number as listed in section 10 of this framework, boxes 6-8.
† Refers to the indicator number in the WHO document titled, *Monitoring and reporting on the health sector's response towards universal access to HIV/AIDS treatment, prevention, care and support 2007-2010*. Available from: http://www.who.int/hiv/universalaccess2010/UAframework_Final%202Nov.pdf

REFERENCES

(Endnotes)

1. *Interim policy on collaborative TB-HIV activities.* Geneva, World Health Organization, 2004.
2. *Tuberculosis control in the Western Pacific Region: 2007 report.* Manila, WHO Regional Office for the Western Pacific, 2007.
3. *Tuberculosis and HIV: a framework to address TB-HIV co-infection in the Western Pacific Region.* Manila, WHO Regional Office for the Western Pacific, 2004.
4. Op cit. Ref 1.
5. *A guide to monitoring and evaluation for collaborative TB/HIV activities.* Geneva, World Health Organization 2004.
6. Op cit. Ref 2
7. Op cit. Ref 2.
8. Op cit. Ref 2.
9. *AIDS epidemic update: December 2007.* Geneva, UNAIDS, 2007.
10. Ibid.
11. *Report on HIV sentinal surveillance in Cambodia*: Phnom Penh, Ministry of Health, National Center for HIV/AIDS, Dermatology and STDs,2003.
12. Op cit. Ref 9.
13. Chan R, Kavi AR, Carl G. HIV and men who have sex with men: perspectives from selected Asian countries. *AIDS,* 1998,12(suppl):59-68.
14. Unpublished data. WHO
15. Op cit. Ref 1.
16. Dye C, et al, for the WHOGSaMP. Global burden of tuberculosis: estimated incidence, prevalence, and mortality by country. *Journal of the American Medical Association,* 1999, 282(7):677-686.
17. Del Amo J, et al. Does tuberculosis accelerate the progression of HIV disease? Evidence from basic science and epidemiology. *AIDS,* 1999;13(10):1151-1158.
18. Ansari NA, et al. Pathology and causes of death in a group of 128 predominantly HIV-positive patients in Botswana, 1997-1998. *International journal of tuberculosis and lung disease,* 2002, 6(1):55-63.
19. Greenberg AE, et al. Autopsy-proven causes of death in HIV-infected patients treated for tuberculosis in Abidjan, Cote d'Ivoire. *AIDS,* 1995, 9(11):1251-1254.
20. Rana FS, et al. Autopsy study of HIV-1-positive and HIV-1-negative adult medical patients in Nairobi, Kenya. *Journal of acquired immune deficiency syndromes,* 2000, 24(1):23-29
21. Op cit. Ref 2.
22. Kalou M, et al. Changes in HIV RNA viral load, CD4+ T-cell counts, and levels of immune activation markers associated with anti-tuberculosis therapy and cotrimoxazole prophylaxis among HIV-infected tuberculosis patients in Abidjan, Cote d'Ivoire. *Journal of medical virology,* 2005, 75(2):202-208.

23. Morris L, *et al*. Human immunodeficiency virus-1 RNA levels and CD4 lymphocyte counts, during treatment for active tuberculosis, in South African patients. *Journal of infectious diseases,* 2003, 187(12):1967-1971.
24. Wiktor SZ, *et al*. Efficacy of trimethoprim-sulphamethoxazole prophylaxis to decrease morbidity and mortality in HIV-1-infected patients with tuberculosis in Abidjan, Cote d'Ivoire: a randomised controlled trial. *Lancet,* 1999, 353(9163):1469-1475.
25. Heller T, *et al*. *Tuberculosis as a late complication of HIV infection in Banteay Meanchey, Cambodia*. Paper presented at: Union World Conference Against Lung Disease, Paris, France, 2006.
26. Nissapatorn V, *et al*. Tuberculosis in HIV/AIDS patients: a Malaysian experience. *Southeast Asian journal of tropical medicine and public health,* 2005, 36(4):946-953.
27. Akksilp S, *et al*. Antiretroviral therapy during tuberculosis treatment and marked reduction in death rate of HIV-infected patients, Thailand. *Emerging infectious disease,* 2007, 13(7):1001.
28. Manosuthi W, *et al*. Survival rate and risk factors of mortality among HIV/tuberculosis-coinfected patients with and without antiretroviral therapy. *Journal of acquired immune deficiency syndromes,* 2006, 43(1):42-46.
29. Varma JK, *et al*. Evaluating the potential impact of the new Global Plan to Stop TB: Thailand, 2004-2005. *Bulletin of the World Health Organization,* 2007, 85(8):586-592.
30. *Op cit*. Ref 28.
31. *Op cit*. Ref 25.
32. Bwire R, Nagelkerke NJ, Borgdorff MW. Finding patients eligible for antiretroviral therapy using TB services as entry point for HIV treatment. *Tropical medicine and international health,* 2006, 11(10):1567-1575.
33. *Op cit*. Ref 27.
34. *Op cit*. Ref 28.
35. Cain KP, *et al*. Epidemiology of HIV-associated tuberculosis in rural Cambodia. *International journal of tuberculosis and lung disease,* 2007, 11(9):1008-1013.
36. Quy H, *et al*. Treatment outcomes by drug resistance and HIV status among tuberculosis patients in Ho Chi Minh City, Vietnam. *International journal of tuberculosis and lung disease,* 2006, 10(1):45-51.
37. Trinh TT, *et al*. HIV-associated TB in An Giang Province, Vietnam, 2001-2004: epidemiology and TB treatment outcomes. *PLoS ONE,* 2007, 2:e507.
38. Mukadi YD, Maher D, Harries A. Tuberculosis case fatality rates in high HIV prevalence populations in sub-Saharan Africa. *AIDS,* 2001, 15(2):143-152.
39. *Guidance on provider-initiated HIV testing and counselling in health facilities.* Geneva, World Health Organization, 2007.
40. *Integrated Management of Adolescent and Adult Illness.* Geneva, World Health Organization, 2006.
41. *Strategic and Technical Advisory Group for Tuberculosis. Seventh meeting. Report on conclusions and recommendations.* Geneva, World Health Organization, 2007.
42. *Ibid.*
43. *Guidelines for HIV surveillance among tuberculosis patients (second edition).* Geneva, World Health Organization, 2004.

44 *Ibid.*
45 *Ibid.*
46 *Op cit.* Ref 35.
47 Kong BN, *et al.* Opportunistic infections and HIV clinical disease stage among patients presenting for care in Phnom Penh, Cambodia. *Southeast Asian journal of tropical medicine and public health,* 2007, 38(1):62-68.
48 *Op cit.* Ref 43.
49 *Global tuberculosis control: surveillance, planning, financing. WHO report 2007.* Geneva, World Health Organization, 2007.
50 *Ibid.*
51 *Op cit.* ref 39.
52 *Op cit.* Ref 49.
53 Centers for Disease Control and Prevention. Unpublished data.
54 Kanara N, *et al. Association between distance to HIV testing site and uptake of HIV testing for tuberculosis patients in Cambodia.* Paper presented at: 1st Union Asia Pacific Region Conference, Kuala Lumpur, Malaysia, 2007.
55 Centers for Disease Control and Prevention. Provider-initiated HIV testing and counselling of TB patients--Livingstone District, Zambia, September 2004-December 2006. *MMWR Morbidity and mortality weekly report, 2008,* Mar 21, 57(11):285-289.
56 *Op cit.* Ref 39.
57 *Op cit.* Ref 39.
58 HIV testing and counselling in TB clinical settings: tools. Atlanta GA, Centers for Disease Control and Prevention. Available from: http://www.cdc.gov/nchstp/od/gap/pa_tb_tools.htm.
59 *Op cit.* Ref 39.
60 *Op cit.* Ref 39.
61 *International standards for tuberculosis care (ISTC).* The Hague, Tuberculosis Coalition for Technical Assistance, 2006.
62 Srikantiah P, *et al.* Elevated HIV seroprevalence and risk behavior among Ugandan TB suspects: implications for HIV testing and prevention. *International journal of tuberculosis and lung disease,* 2007, 11(2):168-174.
63 *Improving the diagnosis and treatment of smear-negative pulmonary and extrapulmonary tuberculosis among adults and adolescents: Recommendations for HIV-prevalent and resource-constrained settings.* Geneva, World Health Organization, 2007.
64 *Op cit.* Ref 39.
65 *Op cit.* Ref 39.
66 *Op cit.* Ref 39.
67 *Op cit.* Ref 16.
68 *Op cit.* Ref 35.
69 *Op cit.* Ref 35.
70 *TB/HIV: a clinical manual.* Geneva, World Health Organization, 2004.
71 *Op cit.* Ref 35.

72 Moore D, et al. Prevalence, incidence and mortality associated with tuberculosis in HIV-infected patients initiating antiretroviral therapy in rural Uganda. AIDS, 30 Mar 2007; 21(6):713-719.
73 Op cit. Ref 35.
74 Op cit. Ref 27.
75 Op cit. Ref 28.
76 Op cit. Ref 25.
77 Smith RL, et al. Factors affecting the yield of acid-fast sputum smears in patients with HIV and tuberculosis. Chest, 1994, 106(3):684-686.
78 Harries AD, et al. Management of pulmonary tuberculosis suspects with negative sputum smears and normal or minimally abnormal chest radiographs in resource-poor settings. International journal of tuberculosis and lung disease, 1998, 2(12):999-1004.
79 Mtei L, et al. High rates of clinical and subclinical tuberculosis among HIV-infected ambulatory subjects in Tanzania. Clinical infectious diseases, 2005, 40(10):1500-1507.
80 Swaminathan S, et al. Unrecognised tuberculosis in HIV-infected patients: sputum culture is a useful tool. International journal of tuberculosis and lung disease, 2004, 8(7):896-898.
81 Op cit. Ref 63.
82 Chheng P, et al. Pulmonary tuberculosis among clients visiting a voluntary confidential counselling and testing center, Cambodia. International journal of tuberculosis and lung disease, 2008, 12(3): 54-62.
83 Cain KP, et al. Developing a clinical algorithm to diagnose TB in HIV-infected persons in Asia. Paper presented at: 38th Union World Conference on Lung Health, Cape Town, South Africa, 2007.
84 Shah NS. (Personal communication)
85 Op cit. Ref 70.
86 Op cit. Ref 63.
87 Op cit. Ref 70.
88 Case definition for extensively drug-resistant tuberculosis. Weekly epidemiological record, 2006, 81(42):408.
89 Shah NS, et al. Worldwide emergence of extensively drug-resistant tuberculosis. Emerging infectious diseases, 2007,13(3):380-387.
90 Gandhi NR, et al. Extensively drug-resistant tuberculosis as a cause of death in patients co-infected with tuberculosis and HIV in a rural area of South Africa. Lancet, 2006, 368(9547):1575-1580.
91 Interim recommendations for the surveillance of drug resistance in tuberculosis. Geneva, World Health Organization, 2007.
92 Op cit. Ref 53.
93 Op cit. Ref 41.
94 Op cit. Ref 70.
95 Bucher HC, et al. Isoniazid prophylaxis for tuberculosis in HIV infection: a meta-analysis of randomized controlled trials. AIDS, 1999, 13(4):501-507.

96   Johnson JL, *et al*. Duration of efficacy of treatment of latent tuberculosis infection in HIV-infected adults. *AIDS,* 2001, 15(16):2137-2147.
97   Whalen CC, *et al*. A trial of three regimens to prevent tuberculosis in Ugandan adults infected with the human immunodeficiency virus. Uganda-Case Western Reserve University Research Collaboration. *New England journal of medicine,* 1997, 337(12):801-808.
98   Woldehanna S, Volmink J. Treatment of latent tuberculosis infection in HIV infected persons. *Cochrane database of systematic reviews,* 2004, (1):CD000171.
99   *Op cit*. Ref 70.
100 *Op cit*. Ref 70.
101 Saukkonen JJ, *et al*. An official ATS statement: hepatotoxicity of antituberculosis therapy. *American journal of respiratory and critical care medicine,* 2006, 174(8):935-952.
102 *Op cit*. Ref 28.
103 *Op cit*. Ref 35.
104 *Op cit*. Ref 36.
105 *Op cit*. Ref 63.
106 *Op cit*. Ref 70.
107 *Antiretroviral therapy for HIV infection in adults and adolescents: recommendations for a public health approach.* Geneva, World Health Organization, 2006.
108 *Op cit*. Ref 27.
109 *Op cit*. Ref 28.
110 Heller T, *et al*. *Experience in establishing ART services in rural Cambodia: follow-up of patients eligible for antiretroviral therapy in 2005.* Paper presented at: HIV/AIDS Implementers Meeting, Kigale, Rwanda, 2007.
111 *Op cit*. Ref 107.
112 *Op cit*. Ref 27.
113 *Op cit*. Ref 28.
114 *Op cit*. Ref 25.
115 *Op cit*. Ref 53.
116 *Op cit*. Ref 28.
117 *Op cit*. Ref 107.
118 *Op cit*. Ref 107.
119 *Op cit*. Ref 107.
120 Centers for Disease Control and Prevention. www.cdc.gov/tb.
121 *Op cit*. Ref 107.
122 *Op cit*. Ref 24.
123 Boeree MJ, *et al*. Efficacy and safety of two dosages of cotrimoxazole as preventive treatment for HIV-infected Malawian adults with new smear-positive tuberculosis. *Tropical medicine and international health,* 2005, 10(8):723-733.
124 Grimwade K, *et al*. Effectiveness of cotrimoxazole prophylaxis on mortality in adults with tuberculosis in rural South Africa. *AIDS,* 2005, 19:163-168.

125 Mwaungulu FB, et al. Cotrimoxazole prophylaxis reduces mortality in human immunodeficiency virus-positive tuberculosis patients in Karonga District, Malawi. *Bulletin of the World Health Organization,* 2004, 82(5):854-863.

126 Zachariah R, et al. Voluntary counselling, HIV testing and adjunctive cotrimoxazole reduces mortality in tuberculosis patients in Thyolo, Malawi. *AIDS,* 2003, 17:1053-1061.

127 Louie JK, et al. Opportunistic infections in hospitalized HIV-infected adults in Ho Chi Minh City, Vietnam: a cross-sectional study. *International journal of STD and AIDS,* 2004, 15(11):758-761.

128 Senya C, et al. Spectrum of opportunistic infections in hospitalized HIV-infected patients in Phnom Penh, Cambodia. *International journal of STD and AIDS,* 2003, 14(6):411-416.

129 Archibald LK, et al. Fever and human immunodeficiency virus infection as sentinels for emerging mycobacterial and fungal bloodstream infections in hospitalized patients >/=15 years old, Bangkok. *Journal of infectious diseases,* 1999, 180(1):87-92.

130 *Op cit.* Ref 27.

131 *Op cit.* Ref 53.

132 *Op cit.* Ref 53.

133 *Op cit.* Ref 37.

134 *Tuberculosis infection control in the era of expanding HIV care and treatment.* Geneva, World Health Organization, 2006. Addendum to: WHO guidelines for the prevention of tuberculosis in health care facilities in resource-limited settings. Geneva, World Health Organization, 1999.

135 *Ibid.*

136 *Ibid.*

137 *Op cit.* Ref 39.

138 *Antiretroviral therapy for HIV infection in infants and children: Towards Universal Access.* Geneva, World Health Organization, 2007.

139 *Guidance for national tuberculosis programmes on the management of tuberculosis in children.* Geneva, World Health Organization, 2006.

140 *Ibid.*

141 Revised BCG vaccination guidelines for infants at risk for HIV infection. *Weekly epidemiological record,* 2007, 82(21):193-196.

142 Global Advisory Committee on Vaccine Safety, 29-30 November 2006. *Weekly epidemiological record,* 2007, 82(3):18-24.

143 *Guide to monitoring and evaluation for collaborative TB/HIV activities.* Geneva, World Health Organization, 2004.

144 *Monitoring and evaluation toolkit: HIV/AIDS, tuberculosis and malaria.* 2nd ed. Geneva, Global Fund to Fight AIDA, Tuberculosis and Malaria, 2006.

145 Martin V, et al. Mycobacterium tuberculosis and human immunodeficiency virus co-infection in intravenous drug users on admission to prison. *International journal of tuberculosis and lung disease,* 2000, 4(1):41-46.

146 *Op cit.* Ref 39.

147 *Op cit.* Ref 134.

148 *Anti-tuberculosis drug resistance in the world: fourth global report.* Geneva, World Health Organization, 2008.
149 *Joint UNAIDS statement on HIV prevention and care strategies for drug users.* Geneva, UNAIDS, 2005.
150 Brassard P, *et al*. Yield of tuberculin screening among injection drug users. *International journal of tuberculosis and lung disease,* 2004, 8(8):988-993.
151 Rubinstien EM, Madden GM, Lyons RW. Active tuberculosis in HIV-infected injecting drug users from a low-rate tuberculosis area. *Jourbal of acquired immune deficiency syndromes and human retrovirology,* 1996, 11(5):448-454.
152 *Breaking down barriers: lessons on providing HIV treatment to injecting drug users.* New York, International Harm Reduction Development Program of the Open Society Institute, 2004.
153 Celentano DD, *et al*. Time to initiating highly active antiretroviral therapy among HIV-infected injection drug users. *AIDS,* 2001, 15(13):1707-1715.
154 HIV drug interactions. Available at: www.hiv-druginteractions.org.
155 *HIV/AIDS care and treatment for people who inject drug in Asia and the Pacific: an essential practice guide.* New Delhi and Manila, WHO Regional Offices for South-East Asia and the Western Pacific, 2008.
156 *Ibid.*
157 *Providing comprehensive TB and HIV prevention, treatment and care services for drug users: an integrated approach.* Geneva, World Health Organization, 2008 (in preparation).
158 Kimerling ME, *et al*. Prevalence of pulmonary tuberculosis among HIV-infected persons in a home care program in Phnom Penh, Cambodia. *International journal of tuberculosis and lung disease,* 2002, 6(11):988-994.
159 Suggaravetsiri P, *et al*. Integrated counselling and screening for tuberculosis and HIV among household contacts of tuberculosis patients in an endemic area of HIV infection: Chiang Rai, Thailand. *International journal of tuberculosis and lung disease,* 2003, 7(12 Suppl 3):S424-431.
160 *TB/HIV research priorities in resource-limited settings: report of an expert consultation.* Geneva, World Health Organization, 2005.
161 *Op cit*. Ref 39.
162 *Op cit*. Ref 39.
163 *Op cit*. Ref 39.
164 *Op cit*. Ref 39.
165 *Op cit*. Ref 39.
166 *Op cit*. Ref 58.
167 *Op cit*. Ref 39.
168 *Op cit*. Ref 39.
169 *Op cit*. Ref 39.
170 *Op cit*. Ref 58.
171 *Op cit*. Ref 53.
172 *Op cit*. Ref 39.
173 http://www.r-project.org.